PumpOne®

BACK
STRENGTHENING

FOR HEALTH & FITNESS

DECLAN CONDRON

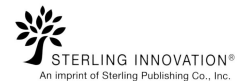

STERLING INNOVATION®
An imprint of Sterling Publishing Co., Inc.

New York / London
www.sterlingpublishing.com

STERLING and the distinctive Sterling logo are registered trademarks of Sterling Publishing Co., Inc.

Library of Congress Cataloging-in-Publication Data
Condron, Declan.
  Back Strengthening for health & fitness / Declan Condron.
    p. cm.
Includes index
ISBN 978-1-4027-5974-1
1. Back exercises. I. Title.
GV508.C69 2008
613.7'1881--dc22
            2008016285

10 9 8 7 6 5 4 3 2 1

Published by Sterling Publishing Co., Inc.
387 Park Avenue South, New York, NY 10016
© 2008 by PumpOne®
Distributed in Canada by Sterling Publishing
c/o Canadian Manda Group, 165 Dufferin Street
Toronto, Ontario, Canada M6K 3H6
Distributed in the United Kingdom by GMC Distribution Services
Castle Place, 166 High Street, Lewes, East Sussex, England BN7 1XU
Distributed in Australia by Capricorn Link (Australia) Pty. Ltd.
P.O. Box 704, Windsor, NSW 2756, Australia

Digital Imaging by Craig Schlossberg
Photography by Susan E. Cohen

Sterling ISBN 978-1-4027-5974-1

For information about custom editions, special sales, premium and corporate purchases, please contact Sterling Special Sales
Department at 800-805-5489 or specialsales@sterlingpublishing.com.

The exercise programs described in this book are based on well-established practices proven to be effective for overall health and fitness, but they are not a substitute for personalized advice from a qualified practitioner. Always consult with a qualified health care professional in matters relating to your health before beginning this or any exercise program. This is especially important if you are pregnant or nursing, if you are elderly, or if you have any chronic or recurring medical condition. As with any exercise program, if at any point during your workout you begin to feel faint, dizzy, or have physical discomfort, you should stop immediately and consult a physician.

The purpose of this book is to educate and is sold with the understanding that the author and the publisher shall have neither liability nor responsibility for any injury caused or alleged to be caused directly or indirectly by the information in this book.

CONTENTS

Introduction ...4

How This Book Works ...8

Safety Precautions ...9

Equipment ...11

Tips for Getting Started ...11

Warming Up and Cooling Down ...12

Warm-ups ...13

LEVEL 1

   Workout 1 ...19

   Workout 2 ...29

   Workout 3 ...39

   Workout 4 ...49

LEVEL 2

   Workout 1 ...59

   Workout 2 ...70

   Workout 3 ...81

   Workout 4 ...92

LEVEL 3

   Workout 1 ...103

   Workout 2 ...114

   Workout 3 ...125

   Workout 4 ...136

Stretch Sequence 1 ...147

Stretch Sequence 2 ...154

Index ...160

INTRODUCTION

Lower back pain is thought to affect as many as 90 percent of Americans at some point in their lives. It is second only to headaches as the most common neurological aliment in the United States, and is a leading cause of missed workdays and job-related disability.

In more than 80 percent of cases, it can be very hard to identify a specific cause of lower back pain. There usually exist a number of symptoms that may result from a variety of causes. Most back pain is the result of either sudden trauma caused by an injury or an accident, or overuse, such as constantly using incorrect posture. Pain levels can vary from a dull muscle ache in one particular region to a stabbing sharp pain that radiates to different areas of the body. The pain may also be accompanied by limited range of motion or movement.

Back pain can be diagnosed as acute if present for less than a month or chronic if it has persisted for longer than that. Acute episodes usually result in some form of physical disability for a number of days. Chronic suffers can experience pain and physical limitations for many years without relief. In the past, the typical approach to back pain was spending a few days in bed and stopping all strenuous activity. Recent studies have shown that this approach may in fact prolong healing.

These days, it is much more common for active rehabilitation to be prescribed as a treatment for back pain. Although no specific back exercises have been found to decrease pain or increase function in people with acute back pain, the general recommendation is to resume near to normal activity as soon as possible. Exercise has been shown to help people with chronic back pain return to normal activities sooner. Active exercise is necessary to alleviate current back pain and speed the rehabilitation process and has also been shown to prevent the occurrence of back pain.

PREVENTION

Since back pain is a prominent ailment affecting so many people, prevention is very important. Good ways to prevent back problems are to use better body mechanics and ergonomic techniques for everyday activities, to reduce excess bodyweight, and to engage in a moderate exercise program that focuses on strengthening the body as a whole, with particular attention to the back extensors, abdominal muscles, and hip muscles.

It is essential to perform exercises correctly. Exercising incorrectly may increase the risk of back pain. Major risks are created by using incorrect posture while lifting, squatting, or twisting with an external load; having poor flexibility and muscle elasticity, particularly in the hamstrings, glutes, and hip flexors; and using poor body mechanics while walking, jogging, or playing sports.

It is possible to prevent, or at least drastic-ally reduce, the chances of developing back problems by incorporating a good, progressive exercise program into an overall healthy lifestyle. Exercising correctly is essential to keep the back, as well as the rest of the body, in good working order. Regular exercise not only strengthens bones, muscles, and other soft tissues but also helps distribute nutrients to the intervertebral disks, keeping them healthy and well nourished. The benefits of exercise include increased strength and improved flexibility and range of motion, reducing the risk of injury and minimizing chances for recurrences. If a person who has been exercising reguarly does suffer an episode of back pain, the severity of the injury and the recovery period is usually much reduced.

Each workout in an effective strength-training program should include exercises to target all the body's major muscle groups, paying particular attention to the core muscle groups of the abdomen, upper and lower back, and legs. It should also include some stretching exercises to help improve flexibility and posture.

SPINAL ANATOMY AND FUNCTION

The human back consists of the spine, which is made up of multiple bones called vertebrae; numerous muscles, which run from the neck to the hips; and other soft tissues such as ligaments, tendons, and intervertebral disks, which hold everything together.

The main functions of the spine are to allow for movement, to protect the spinal cord, and to support bodyweight. It consists of up to 33 bones called vertebrae that run from the base of the skull to the pelvis. There are five different regions of the spine, each with a specific number of differently shaped vertebrae that are either fused together or stacked on top of each other. In the three areas that have stacked vertebrae, each region has a specific shape or curvature that allows for maximum range of motion and shock absorption. Each of these stacked vertebrae also has an open space through which the spinal cord runs. Between each vertebrae are also cartilaginous pads called intervertebral disks. These spongy disks act as shock absorbers, cushioning the spine against the many forces placed on it during everyday activities.

Running the length of the spine are numerous long thin muscles called the erector spinae. These muscles run up and down the spine, connecting the vertebrae and allowing movement in all three planes. Other larger muscles, such as the rectus abdominus, quadratus lumborum, obliques, latissimus dorsi, and ilio-psoas, form a corset around the spine, supporting it and helping it to maintain a neutral position during lifting movements. All these muscles act in synergy to stabilize, move, resist movement, protect, and lend support to produce the best movement possible.

Holding everything together are other soft tissues, including ligaments, which connect bone to bone; tendons, which connect muscle to bone; and intervertebral disks, which cushion the vertebrae and prevent damage to the bones. A large majority of back problems result from injury or degeneration of these disks. With age and overuse, the disks can lose their flexibility and fluidity, reducing their ability to act as shock absorbers and cushion the vertebrae.

BENEFITS OF A REGULAR EXERCISE PROGRAM:

INCREASED BONE DENSITY AND MUSCLE TONE

As you age, you typically lose bone density and muscle tone; it is an unfortunate fact of getting older. Loss of bone density, commonly referred to as osteoporosis, is a major cause of fractures, especially in the elderly. Weight-bearing exercises have been shown to dramatically reduce both bone density loss and muscle tone loss, and may even reverse it. Muscle tone refers to the density and contractile properties of the muscle, not necessarily the size. It describes muscle density and strength.

IMPROVEMENTS IN COORDINATION AND PROPRIOCEPTION

As the brain communicates with the muscles, the muscles talk back to the brain. This response is called proprioception, or sometimes kinesthesia. Muscles sense where your limbs are in space and signal your brain: "your left arm is above your head," or "your right leg is straight out in front." Strength training challenges proprioception and improves the message pathways between the brain and muscles.

DEVELOP BETTER MUSCLE SYNERGY

No muscle group works by itself. Muscle groups work together to facilitate movement and to stabilize and support inert body parts. For example, during a biceps curl, your biceps muscles contract to move your arm, while your deltoid muscles help the movement and also stabilize your shoulder. Meanwhile the triceps muscles work to control the speed of the movement. A properly executed strength-training program can help develop better synergy between muscle groups.

VARIETY

Our bodies are very smart machines. When we want to move, our brain figures out the easiest, most effecient way to do it. When we perform a movement again and again, it becomes easier. Changing the movement slightly gives our bodies a challenge: figuring out a better way to meet the new requirements. A progressive exercise program offers such variety by changing the workouts periodically, giving the body new stimuli and forcing it to adapt and accommodate to them.

HOW THIS BOOK WORKS

This book provides a step-by-step progressive exercise plan. Like a personal trainer, it is a guide to what exercises to perform, in which order, using what level of intensity. It will indicate when to advance to a new level to keep you working toward a stronger, fitter body.

The book is divided into three levels of difficulty, each containing four workouts. Level one workouts contain seven different strength-training exercises and three specific stretches. Levels two and three contain eight different strength-training exercises and three specific stretches. The strength-training exercises target the major muscle groups for a total-body workout each time.

Workouts can be performed at different intensities by varying the number of repetitions and sets, the load used, and the amount of rest between sets. This book offers two different intensity tracks for each workout: the strength track and the tone track. The strength track concentrates on building strength and reducing abdominal weight; the tone track concentrates on defining muscles. There is some crossover between tracks. If you are on the strength track, you will also see increases in muscle tone and definition; on the toning track, you might also gain strength and lose weight.

The three levels provide an exercise plan that becomes more difficult as you get fitter and stronger. We suggest beginning at level one and working your way up to level three, even if you are already experienced with workouts. Level three workouts can be very challenging and may take some time to master, so take your time and enjoy the journey.

For best results, try to do two to three workout sessions per week. Just as the body needs variety, it also needs consistency. Perform each workout a few times in each level before moving forward. Spend a number of weeks rotating through the workouts in level one before attempting levels two and three.

SAFETY PRECAUTIONS

In any exercise program, safety is of the utmost importance. This book is designed to help you prevent injuring your back or to recover from a recurring back problem. The last thing you want is to injure yourself trying to get into better shape and improve your health. Before you start any exercise program, we recommend you do the following:

TALK TO YOUR DOCTOR

Always consult your doctor before starting a fitness program, especially if you have or have had a chronic medical condition, are taking any medications, or are pregnant. Immediately stop exercising if you feel pain, faintness, dizziness, or shortness of breath. Wait awhile. You may decide to quit for the day or to resume slowly.

If you have a preexisting back condition, make sure to get clearance from your physician, physical therapist, or orthopedist before beginning these workouts. You may want to show your physician this book to get his or her opinion. The workouts in this book are designed to build an overall strong body with a focus on a strong core and back to help prevent back problems. It is not a cure for an existing back condition or a replacement of a prescribed therapy program.

GET EQUIPPED

If you are performing these exercises at a gym, be sure to get proper instruction on all equipment before beginning. Most gyms have staff members available to answer questions and give basic instructions. If you are exercising at home, check your equipment to make sure it is in good working order. Read all warnings and instructions on the proper use and maintenance of all equipment before you begin.

MAKE ROOM

Make sure you have enough space to exercise, and avoid exercising on slippery surfaces. Be aware of the surrounding area, other people, and any obstacles that might cause a fall.

SUIT UP

Wear appropriate exercise clothing that is neither too baggy nor too tight. It's a good idea to layer clothing so you can take off a piece of clothing as you gradually get warmer. Be sure to wear some form of footwear, such as comfortable sneakers with a nonslip sole. The facility you are using may have regulations on appropriate clothing.

WARM UP AND COOL DOWN

Always warm up for at least five minutes before starting any workout. Warming up gets the body ready to exercise by increasing its core temperature and muscle elasticity. There are sample warm-up exercises provided in the book. Also, be sure to cool down and stretch after your workout. This will help relax your muscles and return them to their resting length, and allow your core temperature to return to normal. We have included a number of specific stretches for each workout and two individual stretching sessions

that can be performed anytime and anywhere. Flexibility is a very important component of any prevention program.

HAVE WATER ON HAND

It's a good idea to eat something at least two hours before exercising and to have water on hand while you are working out. Be sure to sip water regularly during rest intervals. After working out, replenish your body's energy supplies with a good healthy meal. Take time to rest, relax, and recover.

TAKE IT GRADUALLY

Be sure to follow the progression of exercises in this book. Go at your own pace, taking care not to overdo it. As you get stronger, you can gradually increase the weights you are using. One of the major reasons people drop an exercise program is that they begin too quickly and do not see results as fast as they would like. Progress takes time and patience, and exercise should become a part of your life.

EQUIPMENT

The workouts in this book require the use of various pieces of equipment such as barbells, dumbbells, cable systems, a Swiss ball, a body toning bar, and an exercise mat. These workouts are best performed in a health club or gym setting. They can also be performed in a home gym setting if you have the appropriate equip-ment. In a home gym, elastic tubing can be used as a substitute for cables in cable-system exercises.

Before beginning these workouts, get proper instruction on how to use all the required equipment. If necessary, ask a trainer to help you find the equipment, set it up, and learn how to use it.

TIPS FOR GETTING STARTED

Once you have consulted your doctor, you are ready to get started. You are eager to hit the gym and perform those first repetitions. Consider a few last tips before you begin.

If this is your first time beginning an exercise program, or if it's been a while, take some time to get familiar with the exercises, the required intensity, and particularly the amount of weights you use. Take it very easy at first. You can always increase the intensity as you get stronger and fitter. Gym staff are usually available to answer questions and give basic instructions on setup and use of equipment. If you have specific questions about any exercise or equipment or want alternate exercises using different equipment, e-mail us at Trainer@PumpOne.com.

Once familiar with the exercises and equipment, you are ready to start working out. Be sure to concentrate on breathing as you exercise. Whether you breathe in or out as you lift weights is not as important as remembering to breathe. Never hold your breath.

WARMING UP AND COOLING DOWN

A warm-up is a crucial part of any exercise program. The importance of a structured warm-up can not be overstated. It is essential to get the body ready for activity and help prevent injury. Warming up before working out prepares you for strenuous activity by increasing the temperature of both your core and your muscles. Increasing the temperature helps to loosen muscles, making them more supple and flexible.

A warm-up also increases your heart rate and the rate of blood flow to your muscles, increasing the amount of oxygen and nutrients delivered to them and helping to prepare them and other tissues for activity.

A concise warm-up should last 10 to 15 minutes. It should target all areas of the body, starting with gentle activity such as light cardiovascular work. It should gradually increase in intensity, building up to the exercises in these workouts. Static stretching before working out is optional. We have provided a number of specific stretches for the legs, hips, and back.

Just as important as a warm-up before exercising is a good cool-down afterward. Cooling down lets your core temperature return to normal and helps your muscles relax and return to their original state. Stretching is an integral part of any exercise program. It can help to increase muscle and joint range of motion, which will improve flexibility and may reduce muscle soreness. A major contributor to chronic back pain is inflexibility caused by tight muscles, especially in the hips, glutes, and hamstrings.

We have provided stretches at the end of each workout along with two individual stretching workouts that will target the major muscle groups used.

ELLIPTICAL MACHINE (OR CROSSTRAINER)

- Stand upright on an elliptical machine.

- Pedal forward with your legs to push the foot-pads while pushing and pulling the handles with your arms.

- Perform for 5 to 7 minutes at a moderate intensity.

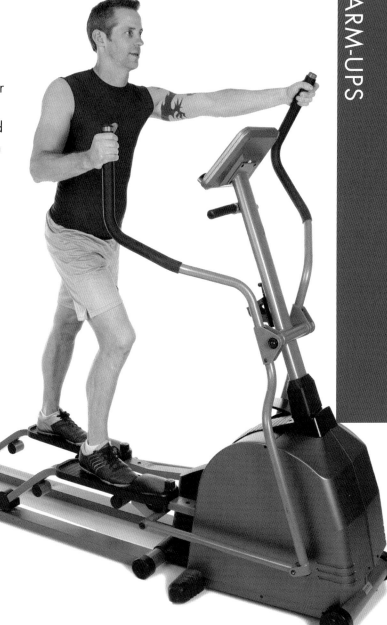

TWISTING PUNCH

- Stand upright facing forward with your hands at chest height.

- Turn to one side, twisting at the hips and shoulders, and punching one arm straight out.

- Turn to the other side and punch out the other arm.

- Perform 2 sets of 20 repetitions in each direction.

JOG IN PLACE

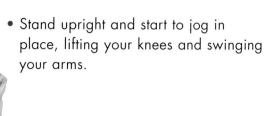

- Stand upright and start to jog in place, lifting your knees and swinging your arms.

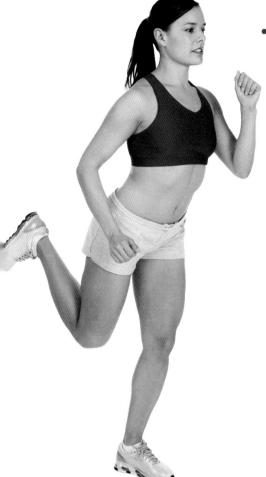

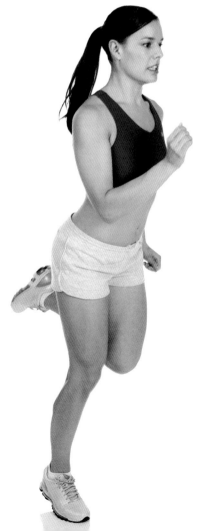

- Try to remain in one spot as you perform the exercise.

- Jog for 3 to 5 minutes at a moderate intensity.

BODYWEIGHT SQUATS

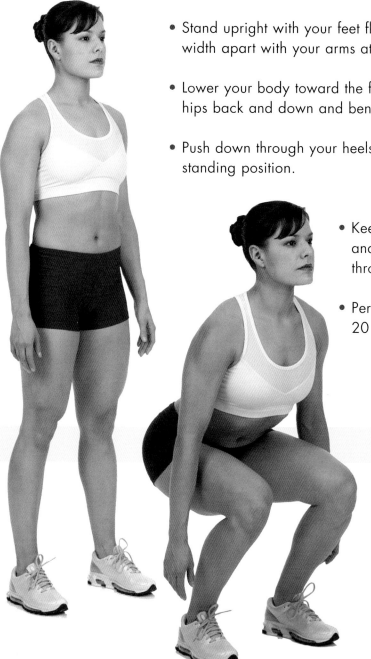

- Stand upright with your feet flat and shoulder-width apart with your arms at your sides.

- Lower your body toward the floor, pushing your hips back and down and bending your knees.

- Push down through your heels to return to standing position.

- Keep your back flat and your head up throughout the exercise.

- Perform 3 sets of 20 reps.

BENCH TOE TAPS

- Start with one foot on a low bench. Lean slightly forward.

- Rapidly switch feet, tapping your toes on the bench with each step.

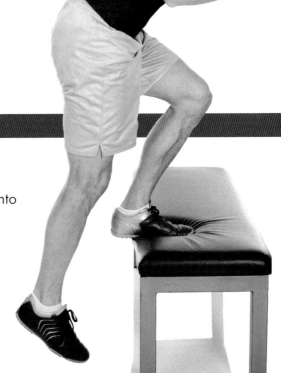

- Make sure to get your top foot onto the bench every time.

- Perform 2 sets of 20 repetitions in each direction.

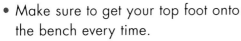

JUMPING JACKS

- Take position: Stand upright with your arms by your sides and your feet together.

- Jump off the floor, bringing your arms straight up to shoulder height and splitting your feet.

- Finish with your arms straight up overhead and your feet about shoulder-width apart.

- Perform 50 reps.

#1 BODYWEIGHT SQUAT

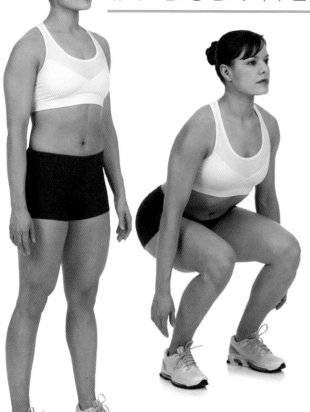

- Stand upright with your feet flat and shoulder-width apart with your arms at your sides.

- Lower your body toward the floor, pushing your hips back and down and bending your knees.

- Push down through your heels to return to standing position.

HINTS

• Back position is very important in all squatting exercises. Always maintain a neutral position. Do not round your lower back or over-arch it. • Keep your head up, looking straight forward with your shoulders back. This will help prevent rounding your upper back.

STRENGTH INTENSITY	TONE INTENSITY
3 sets	2 sets
15 reps	20 reps
45 seconds rest between sets	30 seconds rest between sets

#2 CLOSE-GRIP CABLE PULLDOWN

- Grasp the cable handle with both hands, using a close grip with your arms extended straight over-head.

- Pull the handle down in front to the top of your chest.

- Straighten your arms, returning the handle to the up position.

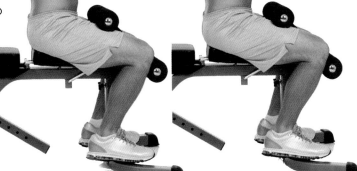

STRENGTH INTENSITY	TONE INTENSITY
3 sets	2 sets
15 reps	20 reps
45 seconds rest between sets	30 seconds rest between sets

HINTS

• Sit upright and do not sway back and forth as you pull the cable handle down.
• Pull down to the point where your elbows are at your sides. • Be sure to go through a full range of motion in the top position, allowing your shoulders to come up to your ears.

#3 PELVIC LIFT

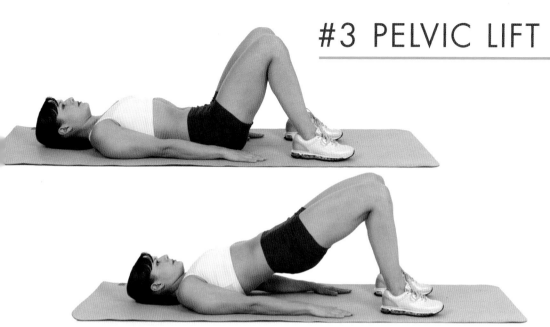

STRENGTH INTENSITY	TONE INTENSITY
3 sets	2 sets
15 reps	20 reps
45 seconds rest between sets	30 seconds rest between sets

- Lie on your back with your knees bent, feet flat, and arms at your sides.

- Lift your hips off the floor until your knees, hips, and shoulders form a straight line.

- Hold this position for ten seconds. Lower your hips back to the floor.

HINTS

• This is a small movement. Do not try to overdo it or force it. • Avoid using your arms to push or hold yourself up. • Control your movement and do not overextend your hips in the top position.

#4 KNEELING PUSH-UP

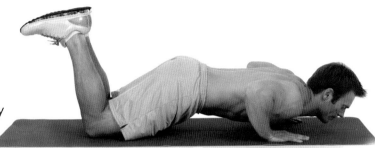

- Support your body on your knees and hands with your elbows bent, feet up, and chest nearly touching the floor.

- Push up to a straight-arm position.

- Keep your hips in line with your head as you bend your elbows to lower yourself back to the floor.

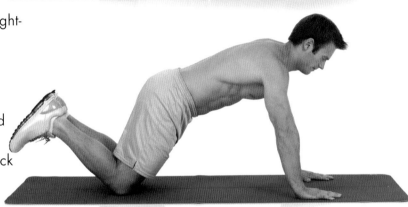

HINTS

• Start with your feet and shins on the floor to add stability. To increase the difficulty, lift your feet off the floor so you are resting on your knees. • Keep your upper body straight as you perform the exercise. Do not let your midsection sag or dip.

STRENGTH INTENSITY	TONE INTENSITY
3 sets	2 sets
15 reps	20 reps
45 seconds rest between sets	30 seconds rest between sets

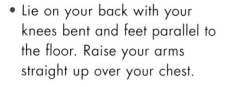

- Lie on your back with your knees bent and feet parallel to the floor. Raise your arms straight up over your chest.

- Lower one leg and the opposite arm overhead, straight down to the floor.

- Return your arm and leg to the mid-position and repeat with the opposite arm and leg.

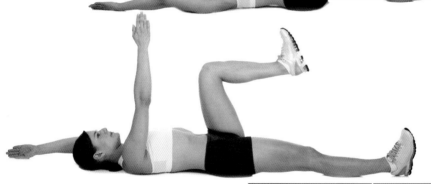

HINTS

• Press your lower back into the floor during the exercise. • Keep the limbs that are not moving as steady as possible during each rep. • Use smooth, controlled motion. Avoid throwing your legs or arms up off the floor.

STRENGTH INTENSITY	TONE INTENSITY
3 sets	2 sets
15 reps	20 reps
45 seconds rest between sets	30 seconds rest between sets

#6 FLYER

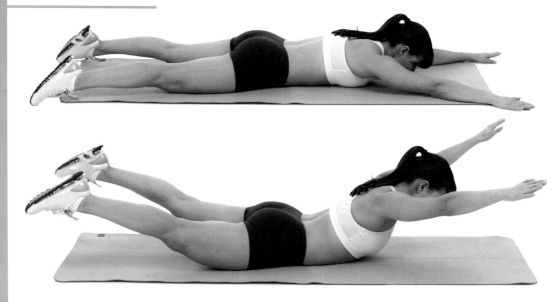

- Lie face down on the floor with your legs straight and your arms stretched out overhead.

- Lift your upper body, arms, and legs together, to about 18 inches off the floor, as if you were flying.

- Hold this position for ten seconds. Then lower yourself back to the floor and repeat.

STRENGTH INTENSITY	TONE INTENSITY
3 sets	2 sets
15 reps	20 reps
45 seconds rest between sets	30 seconds rest between sets

HINTS

• Use controlled movements. Avoid throwing yourself up off the floor. • Lift both your legs and arms to the same height, and keep your head steady throughout. • Do not overextend your lower back. Press your pelvis into the floor to prevent this.

#7 LOWER BODY TWIST

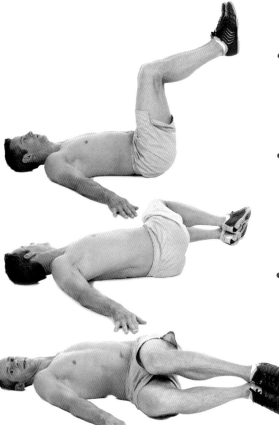

- Lie on your back with your knees bent into a 90-degree angle and your feet lifted, hands at your sides.

- Roll your hips and legs to one side, touching your knee to the floor. Keep your knees bent with your feet together and your upper body stable.

- Then roll your hips and legs to the opposite side to touch the other knee to the floor.

HINTS

- Twist through your midsection, using your abdominal muscles to perform the movement. • Keep your shoulders and your upper back on the floor throughout.

STRENGTH INTENSITY	TONE INTENSITY
3 sets	2 sets
15 reps	20 reps
45 seconds rest between sets	30 seconds rest between sets

#8 GLUTE STRETCH 1

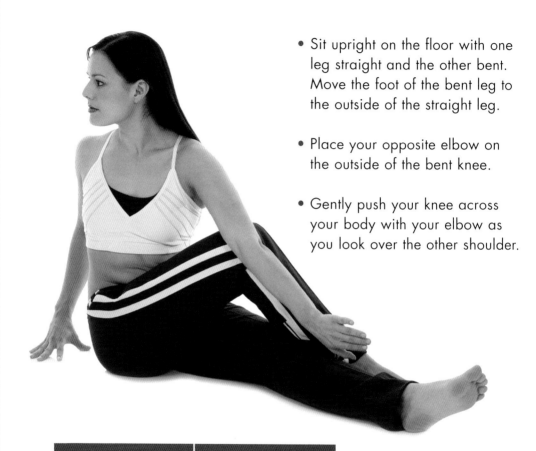

- Sit upright on the floor with one leg straight and the other bent. Move the foot of the bent leg to the outside of the straight leg.

- Place your opposite elbow on the outside of the bent knee.

- Gently push your knee across your body with your elbow as you look over the other shoulder.

STRENGTH INTENSITY	TONE INTENSITY
Hold for 10 seconds. Repeat 3 times on each leg.	Hold for 10 seconds. Repeat 3 times on each leg.

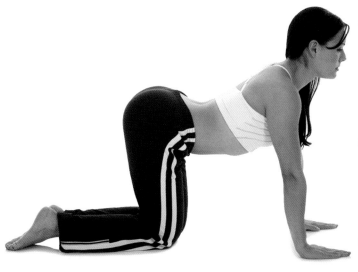

- Position yourself on your hands and knees with your back slightly dropped and your head up, looking forward.

- Round and lift your back by pulling your abdominal muscles in and raising your shoulders.

- Lower your head to look down at the floor.

STRENGTH INTENSITY	TONE INTENSITY
Hold for 10 seconds. Repeat 3 times.	Hold for 10 seconds. Repeat 3 times.

#10 SINGLE LEG STRETCH

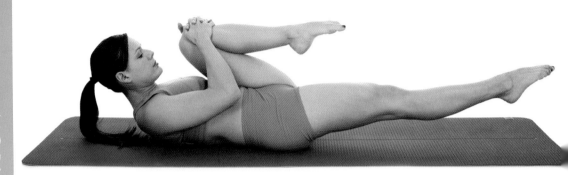

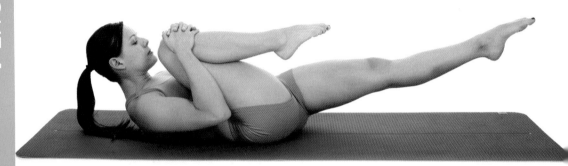

- Lie on your back with your legs straight out and slightly off the floor.

- Slightly raise your head and shoulders off the floor.

- Bring one knee to your chest, grasping at the knee.

- Switch sides.

STRENGTH INTENSITY	TONE INTENSITY
Hold for 10 seconds. Repeat 3 times on each leg.	Hold for 10 seconds. Repeat 3 times on each leg.

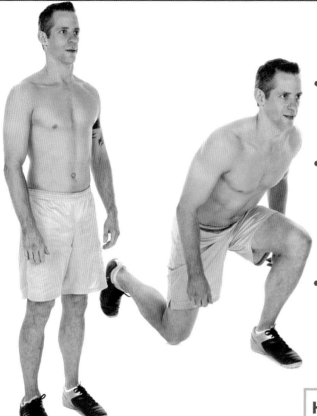

- Stand upright with your arms by your sides, looking straight forward.

- Take a step backward, dropping your back knee to the floor and bending your torso slightly forward with your weight on your front leg.

- Push off your front foot to return to the starting position.

HINTS

- Keep your body weight over your front foot, not on your back foot.
- Lean slightly forward as if you were bending down to set something on the floor in front of you.
- Maintain a flat or neutral spine throughout the exercise.

STRENGTH INTENSITY	TONE INTENSITY
3 sets	2 sets
15 reps	20 reps
45 seconds rest between sets	30 seconds rest between sets

#2 PRONE BENCH ROW

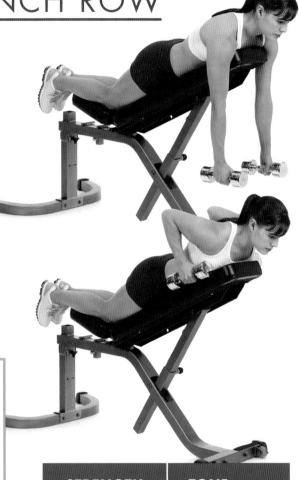

- Position yourself face down on an incline bench, holding dumbbells at your sides with your arms straight and your palms facing in.

- Lift the dumbbells up to the sides of your chest with your elbows moving backward.

- Lower the dumbbells back into the straight-arm position.

HINTS

• As you lift the dumbbells, draw your elbows up along your sides, not outward. • Look down at the floor to keep your head in line with your spine. Do not raise your head as you lift the dumbbells. • Alternate positions are kneeling on the end of the bench with your feet up or sitting with your feet flat on the floor.

STRENGTH INTENSITY	TONE INTENSITY
3 sets	2 sets
15 reps	20 reps
45 seconds rest between sets	30 seconds rest between sets

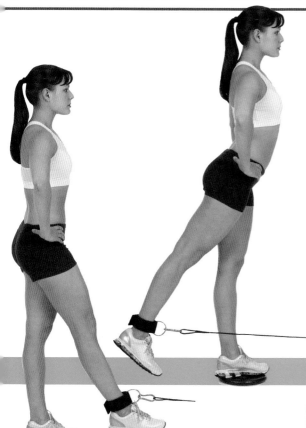

- Stand upright facing a pulley cable system with the cable low and attached to one ankle.

- Place your hands on your hips.

- Draw the attached leg back behind you, keeping your leg straight.

- Use the cable system to maintain your balance, if necessary.

HINTS

• Stand on a small weight plate with your static leg to raise yourself slightly off the floor. This will help prevent dragging your moving foot. • Use smooth, controlled movements, and be careful not to thrust your leg back or pitch your upper body forward.
• Move only through your hips, not your spine.

STRENGTH INTENSITY	TONE INTENSITY
3 sets	2 sets
15 reps	20 reps
45 seconds rest between sets	30 seconds rest between sets

#4 DUMBBELL BENCH PRESS

- Lie on a flat bench holding a dumbbell in each hand at shoulder level with your elbows bent.

- Press the dumbbells up until your arms are straight and the dumbbells are directly over your upper chest.

- Lower the dumbbells by bending at the elbows and returning to the starting position.

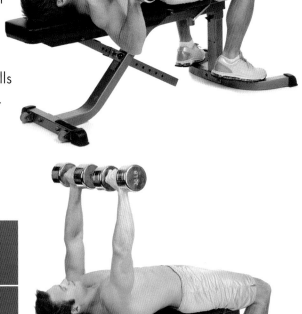

STRENGTH INTENSITY	TONE INTENSITY
3 sets	2 sets
15 reps	20 reps
45 seconds rest between sets	30 seconds rest between sets

HINTS

- Keep the dumbbells directly over your chest. Do not let them wobble outward or inward.
- Do not bang the dumbbells together at the top of the rep. Instead stop them a few inches apart. • Keep your feet flat on the floor throughout the exercise. • Complete a full range of motion, lowering the dumbbells all the way down to your shoulders.

#5 PELVIC TILT

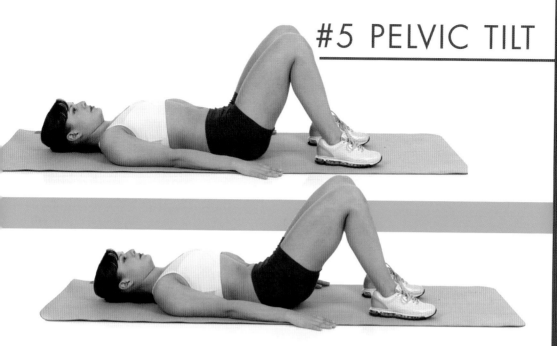

- Lie on your back with your knees bent, feet placed flat, and your arms along your sides.

- Tighten your abdominal muscles by pulling your belly button in and up toward your ribs.

- Press your back into the floor, allowing your pelvis to round slightly.

STRENGTH INTENSITY	TONE INTENSITY
3 sets	2 sets
15 reps	20 reps
45 seconds rest between sets	30 seconds rest between sets

HINTS

• Think about touching your spine with your belly button. • As you round your pelvis slightly, do not lift your hips off the floor. • Breathe smoothly as you perform each rep.

#6 FRONT BRIDGE

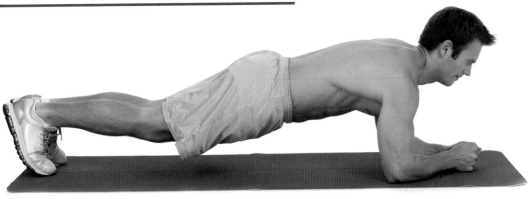

- Lie face down on the floor with your legs straight and arms tucked in by your sides.

- Lift your body off the floor, resting on your toes and forearms. Clasp your hands together to form an inverted V with your forearms.

- Keep your body in a straight line and your back flat.

- Hold for ten seconds, then lower yourself back to the floor and repeat.

HINTS

• Start in a kneeling position with your elbows on the floor. Lift your hips and hold your torso in a straight line throughout the exercise. • Keep your forearms on the floor with your elbows directly under your shoulders. • Start with your feet slightly apart.

STRENGTH INTENSITY	TONE INTENSITY
3 sets	2 sets
15 reps	20 reps
45 seconds rest between sets	30 seconds rest between sets

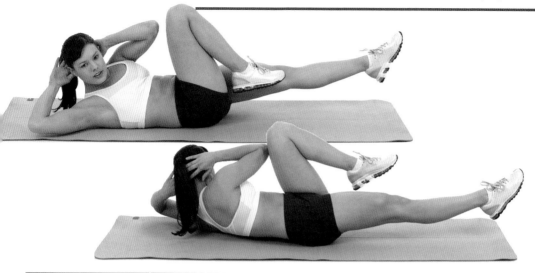

STRENGTH INTENSITY	TONE INTENSITY
3 sets	2 sets
15 reps	20 reps
45 seconds rest between sets	30 seconds rest between sets

- Lie on your back with your legs straight out and your hands at the sides of your head.

- Lift your head and shoulders off the floor, bringing one knee toward your chest.

- Twist your torso, bringing the opposite elbow to your knee.

- Lower your upper body and leg to the floor, and repeat on the opposite side, using your other leg.

HINTS

• Return fully to the down position before switching to the other side. • Turn your head and shoulders as you rotate to each side. • Try to keep your feet off the floor throughout the exercise, but if this is too much stress, touch your heels to the floor.

#8 GLUTE STRETCH 2

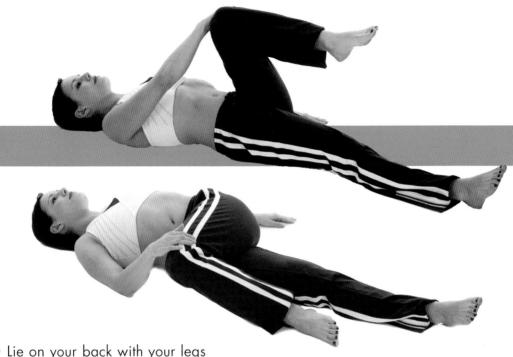

- Lie on your back with your legs straight out.

- Bending at the knee, bring one leg up and across your body.

- Use your opposite hand to pull your knee across and down toward the floor.

STRENGTH INTENSITY	TONE INTENSITY
Hold for 10 seconds. Repeat 3 times on each leg.	Hold for 10 seconds. Repeat 3 times on each leg.

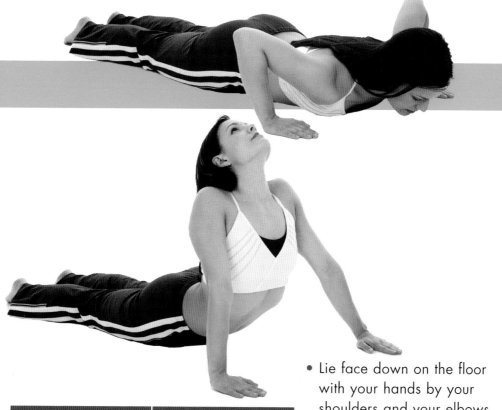

STRENGTH INTENSITY	TONE INTENSITY
Hold for 10 seconds. Repeat 3 times.	Hold for 10 seconds. Repeat 3 times.

- Lie face down on the floor with your hands by your shoulders and your elbows bent.

- Push your upper body up, arching your back, while keeping your hips and legs on the floor. Look upward.

- Try to keep your shoulders in line with your wrists.

#10 HAMSTRING STRETCH 1

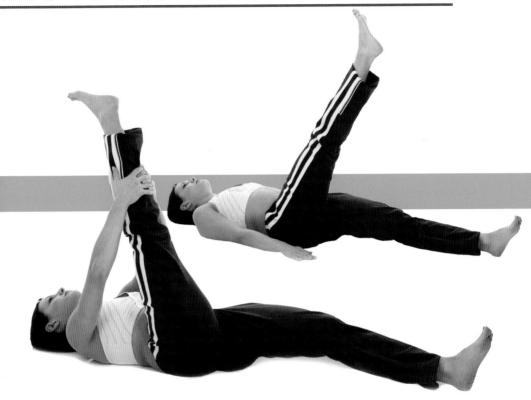

- Lie on your back with both legs straight out on the floor, arms at your side.

- Lift one leg straight up and grasp it behind the calf or ankle. Gently pull the leg toward your head.

- Bend your knee slightly, if necessary.

STRENGTH INTENSITY	TONE INTENSITY
Hold for 10 seconds. Repeat 3 times on each leg.	Hold for 10 seconds. Repeat 3 times on each leg.

#1 DUMBBELL DEADLIFT

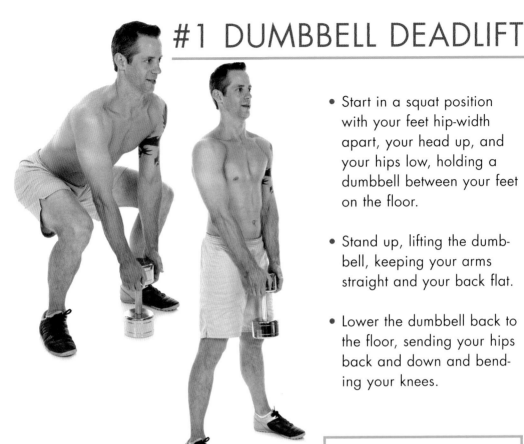

- Start in a squat position with your feet hip-width apart, your head up, and your hips low, holding a dumbbell between your feet on the floor.

- Stand up, lifting the dumbbell, keeping your arms straight and your back flat.

- Lower the dumbbell back to the floor, sending your hips back and down and bending your knees.

HINTS

- Back position is very important in squatting exercises. Keep your back in a neutral position; do not round your lower back or over-arch it. • Hold your head up, looking straight forward, and keep your shoulders back.
- Touch the dumbbell on the floor at the end of each rep.

STRENGTH INTENSITY	TONE INTENSITY
3 sets	2 sets
15 reps	20 reps
45 seconds rest between sets	30 seconds rest between sets

#2 CABLE SEATED ROW

- Sit upright on a bench holding the cable's handle with your arms straight out in front and your back straight and flat.

- Pull the handle straight in to your chest, bending your elbows.

- Slowly extend your arms to return the handle to the starting position.

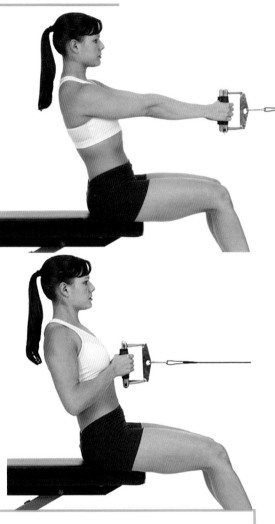

STRENGTH INTENSITY	TONE INTENSITY
3 sets	2 sets
15 reps	20 reps
45 seconds rest between sets	30 seconds rest between sets

HINTS

- As you pull the handle in, lift your chest slightly and pull your shoulder blades together.
- Keep your back upright, and do not sway back and forth as you pull the handle in and out. • Keep your head up, looking straight forward, and do not raise your shoulders. • Your elbows should move backward close to your sides, not outward.

#3 GLUTE BRIDGE

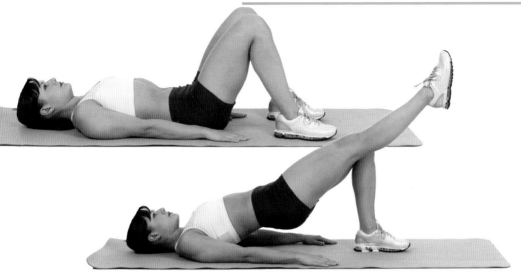

STRENGTH INTENSITY	TONE INTENSITY
3 sets	2 sets
15 reps	20 reps
45 seconds rest between sets	30 seconds rest between sets

- Lie on your back with your knees bent and feet flat on the mat, hands at your sides.

- Straighten and lift one leg, and lift your hips off the floor, making a straight line from your ankle to your shoulder.

- Hold this position for ten seconds. Lower yourself to the floor and repeat on the other side.

HINTS

• This is a small movement; do not overdo it or force it. • Don't use your arms to push and hold yourself up; use your glutes, hamstrings, and abs. • Control the movement; do not thrust your hips into the top position. • Only your head, shoulders, arms, and one foot should contact the floor at the top position.

#4 BENCH DIP

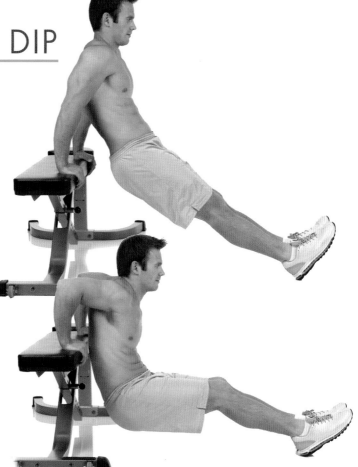

- Place your palms on a bench behind you and set your heels on the floor with your legs and arms straight.

- Bending your elbows, lower your body down toward the floor.

- Push up through your palms, straightening your arms to return to the starting position.

HINTS

• Start by sitting on the bench with your feet on the floor. Position your hands on the edge of the bench.
• Keep your head up, and look straight forward to maintain a neutral back position. • Once you feel comfortable with the exercise, you can dip lower than your elbows to shoulder level.

STRENGTH INTENSITY	TONE INTENSITY
3 sets	2 sets
15 reps	20 reps
45 seconds rest between sets	30 seconds rest between sets

#5 CRUNCH

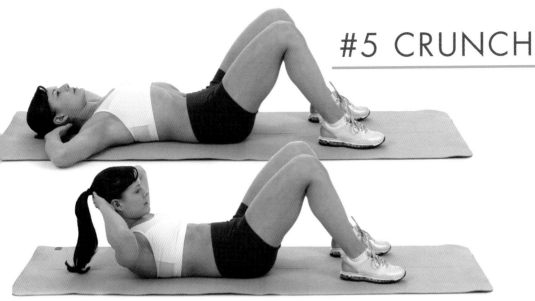

- Lie on your back with your knees bent and feet flat; place your hands at the sides of your head.

- Lift your head and shoulders off the floor, keeping your feet flat.

- Concentrate on contracting your abdominal muscles, not on pulling your head up with your hands.

- Lower your head and shoulders and repeat.

STRENGTH INTENSITY	TONE INTENSITY
3 sets	2 sets
15 reps	20 reps
45 seconds rest between sets	30 seconds rest between sets

HINTS

• Control the movement through your midsection and avoid jerky movements. • Do not use your hands to pull your head and neck up. • Lift just your head and shoulders off the floor, not your whole back. • Start with your feet about shoulder-width apart.

#6 ALTERNATING FLYER

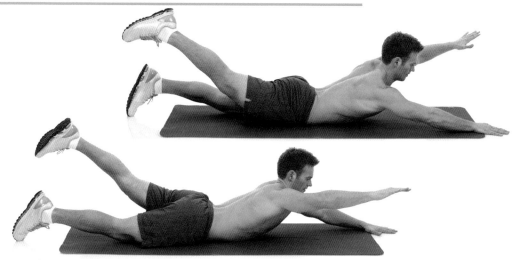

- Lie face down on the floor with your legs straight and your arms outstretched in front.

- Raise one arm and the opposite leg straight up to about 18 inches off the floor.

- Slowly lower both, and repeat with the other arm and leg.

- Be sure to keep your arms and legs straight and your head steady.

STRENGTH INTENSITY	TONE INTENSITY
3 sets	2 sets
15 reps	20 reps
45 seconds rest between sets	30 seconds rest between sets

HINTS

• Use smooth, controlled movements. Avoid jerking yourself up off the floor. • Lift both leg and arm up to the same height and keep your head steady. • Do not lift your head as you raise your arm and leg; keep it in line with your spine.

#7 CABLE TWIST

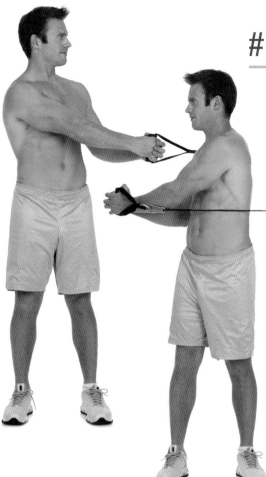

- Stand upright, feet facing forward, upper body turned to one side. Grasp a cable handle with both hands at waist height.

- Twist through your hips to the opposite side, turning your head and shoulders and keeping your arms straight.

- Twist back to the starting side, moving your hips.

HINTS

- Concentrate on moving your hips and shoulders, not your arms.
- Keep your arms straight throughout the exercise. • Turn both your head and shoulders to each side as you perform each rep. • Shift your feet slightly, if necessary.

STRENGTH INTENSITY	TONE INTENSITY
3 sets	2 sets
15 reps	20 reps
45 seconds rest between sets	30 seconds rest between sets

#8 GLUTE STRETCH 3

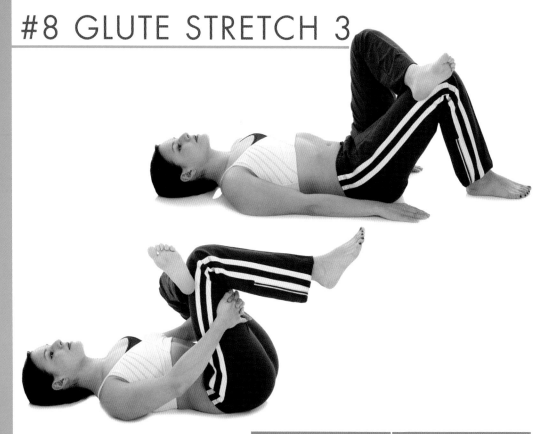

- Lie on your back with one knee bent and your foot flat. Place the ankle of the opposite leg on the bent knee.

- Clasp your hands behind the bottom knee.

- Gently pull the bent knee toward your chest.

STRENGTH INTENSITY	TONE INTENSITY
Hold for 10 seconds. Repeat 3 times on each leg.	Hold for 10 seconds. Repeat 3 times on each leg.

#9 BACK STRETCH 2

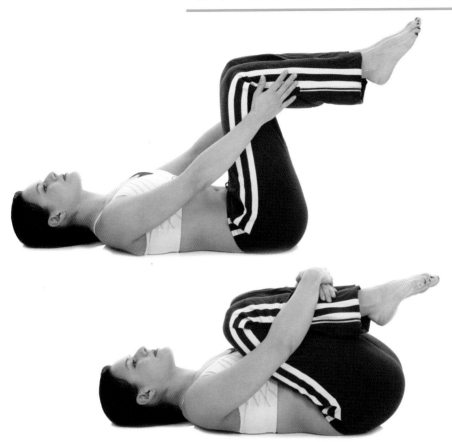

STRENGTH INTENSITY	TONE INTENSITY
Hold for 10 seconds. Repeat 3 times.	Hold for 10 seconds. Repeat 3 times.

- Lie on your back with knees bent to form an angle of 90 degrees. Grasp your knees.

- Gently pull your knees to your chest, allowing your lower back to round slightly.

#10 HIP FLEXOR STRETCH 1

- With one knee on the floor, place the other foot flat on the floor in front of you, forming a 90-degree angle between the knees.

- Lunge forward, shifting your weight onto your front foot and pushing your back hip toward the floor.

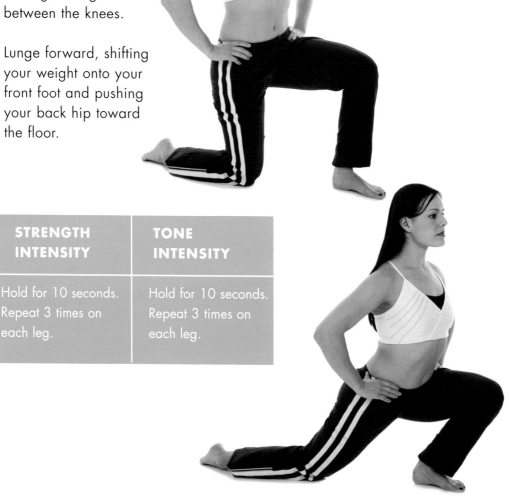

STRENGTH INTENSITY	TONE INTENSITY
Hold for 10 seconds. Repeat 3 times on each leg.	Hold for 10 seconds. Repeat 3 times on each leg.

#1 BODYWEIGHT SIDE LUNGE

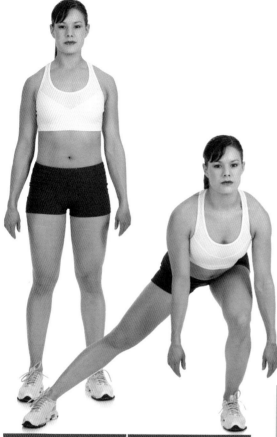

- Stand upright with your arms by your sides and your head up, looking straight forward.

- Step laterally to one side, lowering your body to a half squat and leaning slightly forward with your weight on the outside leg. Keep your trailing leg straight.

- Push off your outside foot to return to the starting position.

- Repeat the exercise on the other leg.

STRENGTH INTENSITY	TONE INTENSITY
3 sets	2 sets
15 reps	20 reps
45 seconds rest between sets	30 seconds rest between sets

HINTS

• Back position is very important in squatting exercises. Keep your back in a neutral position; do not round your lower back or over-arch it. • Keep your head up, looking straight forward, with your shoulders back. • Keep your body weight over your outside foot to help maintain balance and to push with. Keep the other leg straight throughout.

#2 WIDE GRIP PULLDOWN

- Grasp a tension bar using a shoulder-width grip with your arms extended straight overhead.

- Pull the bar down in front to the top of your chest.

- Straighten your arms to return the bar to the up position.

- Sit upright without swaying back and forth.

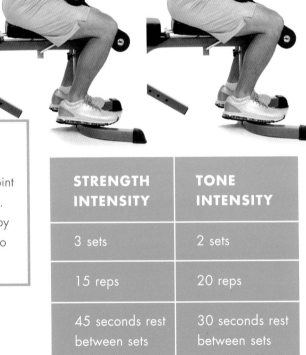

HINTS

- Stay upright and pull down to a point where your elbows are by your sides.
- Complete the full range of motion by allowing your shoulders to come up to your ears at the top of the stretch.

STRENGTH INTENSITY	TONE INTENSITY
3 sets	2 sets
15 reps	20 reps
45 seconds rest between sets	30 seconds rest between sets

#3 CABLE HIP ABDUCTION

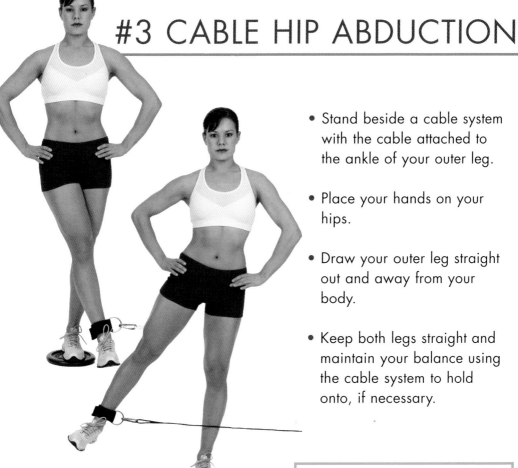

- Stand beside a cable system with the cable attached to the ankle of your outer leg.

- Place your hands on your hips.

- Draw your outer leg straight out and away from your body.

- Keep both legs straight and maintain your balance using the cable system to hold onto, if necessary.

STRENGTH INTENSITY	TONE INTENSITY
3 sets	2 sets
15 reps	20 reps
45 seconds rest between sets	30 seconds rest between sets

HINTS

• With your stable leg, stand on a small weight plate to raise yourself slightly off the floor. This will help stabilize you. • Control your motion, and be careful not to thrust your leg or pitch your upper body sideways. • Move through your hips, not your spine.

#4 DUMBBELL INCLINE BENCH PRESS

- Lie back on an incline bench holding a dumbbell in each hand at shoulder level with your elbows bent.

- Press the dumbbells up until your arms are straight and the dumbbells are directly over your upper chest.

- Lower the dumbbells by bending at the elbows and return to the starting position.

HINTS

- Keep the dumbbells directly over your upper chest. Do not let them move outward or inward. • Do not bang the dumbbells together at the top of each rep. Instead, stop them a few inches apart. • Keep your feet flat on the floor throughout the exercise. • Complete the full range of motion, coming all the way down to your shoulders.

STRENGTH INTENSITY	TONE INTENSITY
3 sets	2 sets
15 reps	20 reps
45 seconds rest between sets	30 seconds rest between sets

#5 FEET-UP CRUNCH

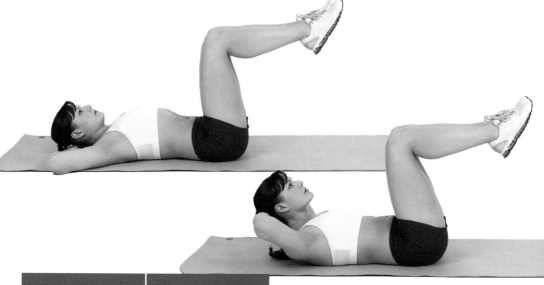

STRENGTH INTENSITY	TONE INTENSITY
3 sets	2 sets
15 reps	20 reps
45 seconds rest between sets	30 seconds rest between sets

- Lie on your back with your knees bent and feet raised, forming a 90-degree angle, and place your hands at the sides of your head.

- Lift your head and shoulders off the floor, keeping your knees bent and your legs steady.

- Concentrate on contracting your abdominal muscles; do not pull your head up with your hands.

- Lower your head and shoulders.

HINTS

- Control the movement through your midsection, and avoid jerky movements. • Lift just your head and shoulders off the floor, not your whole back. • Do not pull your knees in as you raise your head and shoulders.

#6 QUAD FLYER

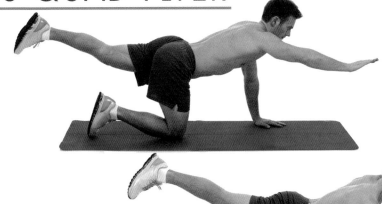

- Position yourself on all fours with both your knees and hands on the floor.

- Raise one arm and the opposite leg straight up to shoulder height.

- Slowly lower your arm and leg. Repeat with the other arm and leg.

- Take your time, and be sure to maintain your balance.

STRENGTH INTENSITY	TONE INTENSITY
3 sets	2 sets
15 reps	20 reps
45 seconds rest between sets	30 seconds rest between sets

HINTS
• Use control to avoid throwing your arm and leg up. • Lift both your legs and arms up to the same height, and keep your head steady. • Do not lift your head as you raise your arm and leg; keep it in line with your spine.

#7 OBLIQUE BRIDGE

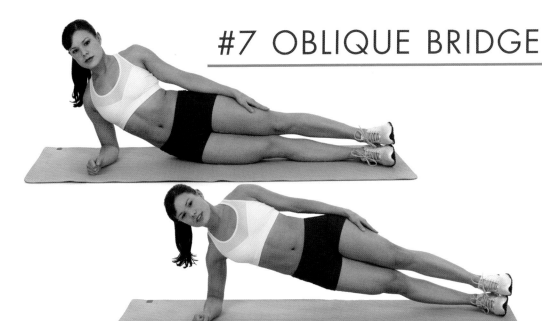

STRENGTH INTENSITY	TONE INTENSITY
3 sets	2 sets
15 reps	20 reps
45 seconds rest between sets	30 seconds rest between sets

- Lie on one side propped up on your elbow and hip, with your legs straight out on top of each other.

- Place your other arm along your side.

- Lift your body off the floor, resting on only your forearm and foot.

- Hold for ten seconds, and then lower yourself back to the floor. Repeat on other side.

HINTS

- Keep your body in a straight line with your elbow directly under your shoulder.
- Keep one foot on top of the other, if possible. • For increased balance, begin with your top hand on the floor.

#8 HAMSTRING STRETCH 2

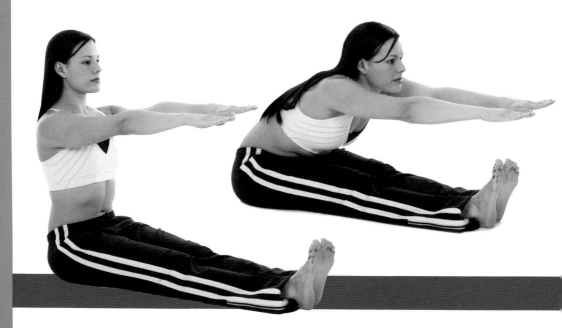

- Sit upright with both your legs and arms straight out in front.

- Reach forward, stretching your arms toward your toes, keeping your legs straight.

STRENGTH INTENSITY	TONE INTENSITY
Hold for 10 seconds. Repeat 3 times.	Hold for 10 seconds. Repeat 3 times.

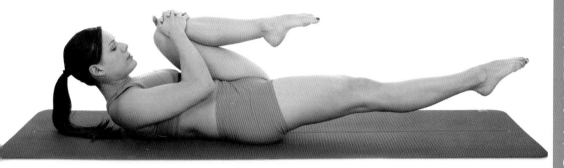

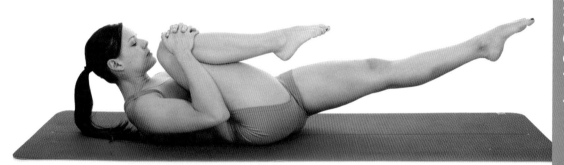

STRENGTH INTENSITY	TONE INTENSITY
Hold for 10 seconds. Repeat 3 times on each leg.	Hold for 10 seconds. Repeat 3 times on each leg.

- Lie on your back with your legs straight out and slightly off the floor.

- Bring one knee in to your chest, holding it at the knee.

- Slightly raise your head and shoulders off floor.

#10 HIP FLEXOR STRETCH 2

- With one knee positioned ahead of you and the other on the floor, move slightly forward into a lunge.

- Lean into your front foot, pushing the back hip toward the floor.

- Raise your back heel to your buttocks and grasp it at your ankle.

- Gently pull your foot closer to your buttocks to feel a greater stretch.

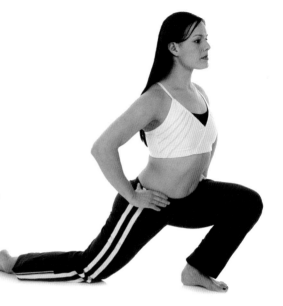

STRENGTH INTENSITY	TONE INTENSITY
Hold for 10 seconds. Repeat 3 times on each leg.	Hold for 10 seconds. Repeat 3 times on each leg.

#1 BODYWEIGHT LUNGE

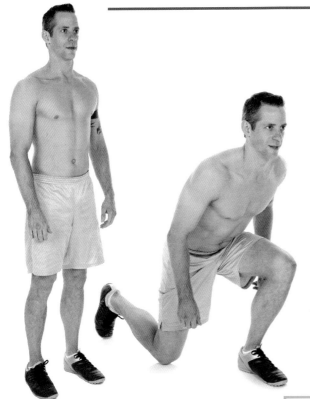

- Stand upright with your arms by your sides and your head up, looking straight forward.

- Take a step forward and drop your back knee toward the floor, bending at the hip and knee.

- Lean slightly forward, keeping all your weight on the front foot.

- Push off the front foot to return to the starting position. Repeat on the other side.

STRENGTH INTENSITY	TONE INTENSITY
3 sets	2 sets
12 reps	15 reps
45 seconds rest between sets	30 seconds rest between sets

HINTS

• Back position is very important in squatting exercises. Keep your back in a neutral position; do not round your lower back or over-arch it.
• Keep your body weight over your front foot. • Lean slightly forward as if you are bending down to put something on the floor in front of you.

#2 DUMBBELL ROW OVER BENCH

- Position yourself over a row bench.

- Holding a dumbbell in one hand with your arm straight, place the opposite knee and hand on the bench. Keep your back flat.

- Bend your elbow to lift the dumbbell up to the side of your chest.

- Lower the dumbbell to the starting position, keeping your back in a neutral position. Repeat on the other arm.

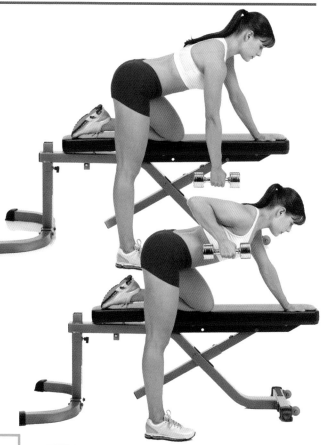

HINTS

- Look toward the floor as you move to maintain a neutral spine. • Do not raise your head as you lift the dumbbell. • Lift the dumbbell so your elbow is by your side and comes above your shoulder.

STRENGTH INTENSITY	TONE INTENSITY
3 sets	2 sets
12 reps	15 reps
45 seconds rest between sets	30 seconds rest between sets

#3 GLUTE BRIDGE MARCH

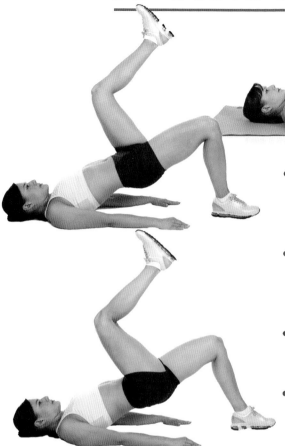

- Lie on your back with your knees bent and your feet flat, placing your hands at your sides.

- Lift your hips off the floor, making a straight line from your knees to your shoulders.

- Now lift one foot high with your knee bent as if you are taking a big step.

- Lower your leg, and repeat on the other side as if you were marching.

STRENGTH INTENSITY	TONE INTENSITY
3 sets	2 sets
12 reps	15 reps
45 seconds rest between sets	30 seconds rest between sets

HINTS

• These are small movements, so don't overdo or force them. • Avoid using your arms to push or hold yourself up. • Use control as you move. Do not thrust your hips up at the top position. • At the top position, only your head, shoulders, arms, and one foot should be in contact with the floor.

#4 PUSH-UP

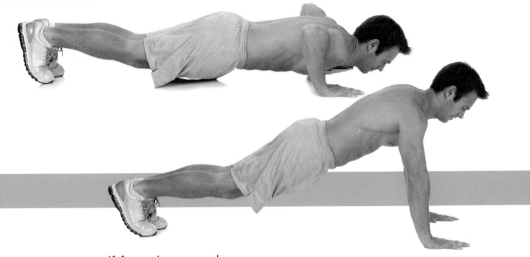

- Position yourself face down on the mat. Support your body on your toes and hands with bent elbows so your chest nearly touches the floor.

- Push up and away to a straight-arm position.

- Lower your body back to the starting position.

- Keep your back flat and your hips in line with your shoulders.

STRENGTH INTENSITY	TONE INTENSITY
3 sets	2 sets
12 reps	15 reps
45 seconds rest between sets	30 seconds rest between sets

HINTS

- Start by lying on your stomach with your hands next to your shoulders. • Drop down till your chest is nearly touching the floor, and push back up to extend your arms fully.
- Look down at the floor to maintain a neutral spine. Do not move your head.

#5 DUMBBELL OVERHEAD PRESS

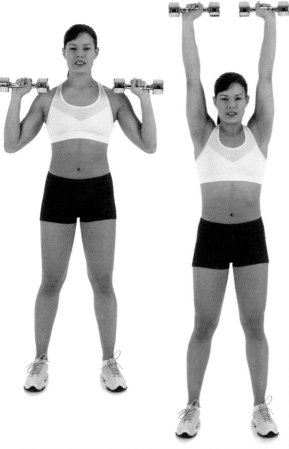

- Stand upright holding a dumbbell in each hand at shoulder height, with your elbows bent and your palms facing forward.

- Press the dumbbells overhead, extending your arms fully.

- Lower the dumbbells to shoulder-level again by bending your elbows.

HINTS

• Keep your back upright by contracting your core muscles as you push the dumbbells overhead. • Go through the full range of motion from shoulder level to arms fully extended overhead and back again. • Start with your feet about shoulder-width apart. To challenge your stability, bring your feet closer together.

STRENGTH INTENSITY	TONE INTENSITY
3 sets	2 sets
12 reps	15 reps
45 seconds rest between sets	30 seconds rest between sets

#6 CRUNCH

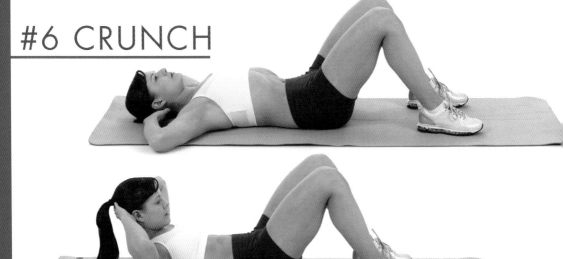

- Lie on your back with your knees bent and your feet flat on the mat. Place your hands at the sides of your head.

- Lift your head and shoulders off the floor, keeping your feet flat.

- Concentrate on contracting your abdominal muscles; do not pull your head up with your hands.

- Lower your head and shoulders back to the floor.

STRENGTH INTENSITY	TONE INTENSITY
3 sets	2 sets
12 reps	15 reps
45 seconds rest between sets	30 seconds rest between sets

HINTS

• Control the movement through your midsection. Avoid jerky movements. • Never use your hands to pull your head and neck up. • Lift only your head and shoulders up off floor, not your whole back.

#7 SWISS BALL Y

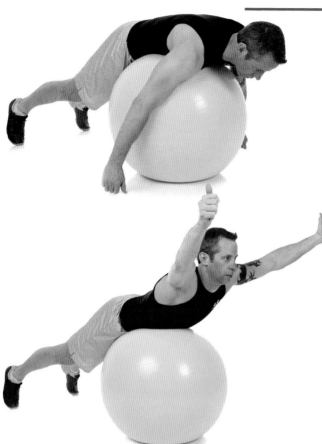

- Lie face down on a Swiss ball, resting on your mid-chest with your feet touching the floor and your arms hanging forward over the ball.

- Raise your upper body off the ball, lifting your arms up straight in front to form a Y with your thumbs up.

- Hold this position for ten seconds. Lower yourself back to the ball.

STRENGTH INTENSITY	TONE INTENSITY
3 sets	2 sets
12 reps	15 reps
45 seconds rest between sets	30 seconds rest between sets

HINTS

- Lift yourself just to the point where your chest is off the ball. • Keep your upper body straight at the top of the movement.
- Do not over-arch your lower back.
- Push your toes into the floor to help keep yourself stable.

#8 DUMBBELL SIDE BEND

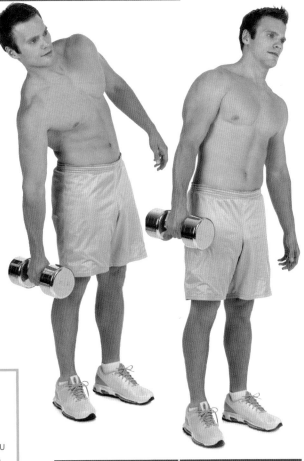

- Stand upright, leaning to one side, grasping a dumbbell with your inside arm held straight.

- Bend to the opposite side, raising the dumbbell.

- Bend back to the starting position, keeping your arm straight throughout.

- Repeat on the opposite arm.

HINTS

• This is a lateral, side-to-side movement. • Do not bend your elbow; you are not trying to lift the dumbbell with your arm. • Bend through your midsection only. Don't bend your hips or knees. • Keep the dumbbell close to your body throughout the exercise.

STRENGTH INTENSITY	TONE INTENSITY
3 sets	2 sets
12 reps	15 reps
45 seconds rest between sets	30 seconds rest between sets

#9 HAMSTRING STRETCH 3

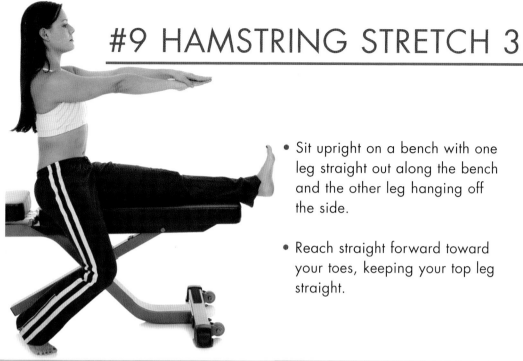

- Sit upright on a bench with one leg straight out along the bench and the other leg hanging off the side.

- Reach straight forward toward your toes, keeping your top leg straight.

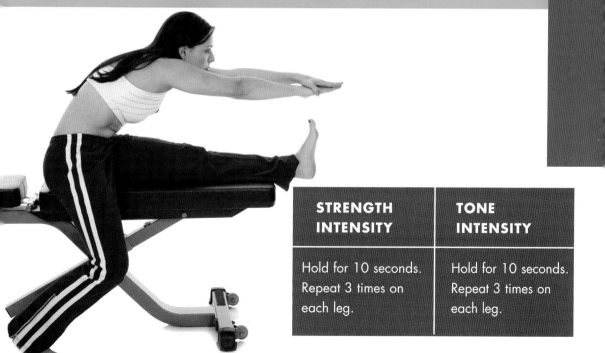

STRENGTH INTENSITY	TONE INTENSITY
Hold for 10 seconds. Repeat 3 times on each leg.	Hold for 10 seconds. Repeat 3 times on each leg.

#10 LATERAL STRETCH

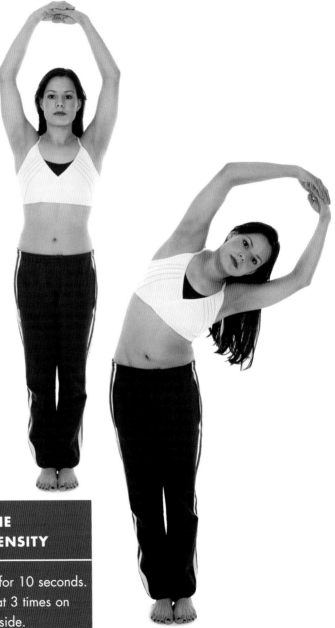

- Stand upright with your feet together and your arms straight up overhead, hands clasped.

- Lean to one side, moving your arms laterally.

- Come back to the upright position and switch sides.

STRENGTH INTENSITY	TONE INTENSITY
Hold for 10 seconds. Repeat 3 times on each side.	Hold for 10 seconds. Repeat 3 times on each side.

#11 HIP FLEXOR STRETCH 1

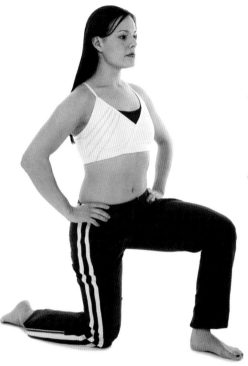

- With one knee on the floor, step slightly forward into a lunge with the other leg.

- Lean into your front foot and push your back hip toward the floor.

STRENGTH INTENSITY	TONE INTENSITY
Hold for 10 seconds. Repeat 3 times on each leg.	Hold for 10 seconds. Repeat 3 times on each leg.

#1 DUMBBELL SPLIT SQUAT

- Stand upright with your feet split front to back, holding a dumbbell in each hand at your sides.

- Keep your head up and look straight forward.

- Lower your body, bending at the hips and knees and leaning slightly forward with your weight on your front leg.

- Push off your front foot to return to the starting position.

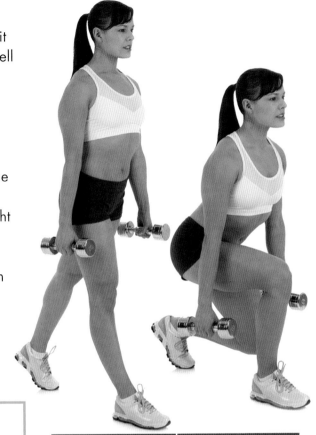

HINTS

• Keep your back in a neutral position; do not round your lower back or over-arch it. • Keep your head up, looking straight forward, with your shoulders back. • Move straight up and down, not forward into your knees.

STRENGTH INTENSITY	TONE INTENSITY
3 sets	2 sets
12 reps	15 reps
45 seconds rest between sets	30 seconds rest between sets

#2 CLOSE-GRIP CABLE PULLDOWN

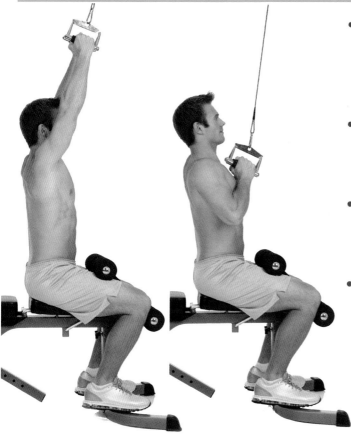

- Grasp a cable handle using a closed grip with your arms extended straight overhead.

- Pull the handle down in front to the top of your chest without swaying.

- Straighten your arms to return the handle to the up position.

- Sit upright and do not sway. Be sure to go through the full range of motion at the top position.

STRENGTH INTENSITY	TONE INTENSITY
3 sets	2 sets
12 reps	15 reps
45 seconds rest between sets	30 seconds rest between sets

HINTS

- Pull down to the point where your elbows are at your sides.
- At the top position, allow your shoulders to come up to your ears.

#3 HIP ABDUCTION WITH BAR

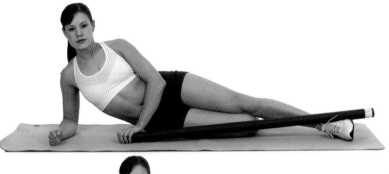

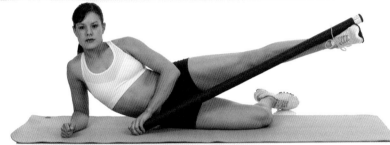

- Lie on your side with your top leg straight and a bar resting across your ankle.

- Raise your leg and the bar straight up. Then, slowly lower your leg and the bar back to the floor.

- Perform all the reps on one side and then switch legs to repeat.

STRENGTH INTENSITY	TONE INTENSITY
3 sets	2 sets
12 reps	15 reps
45 seconds rest between sets	30 seconds rest between sets

HINTS

• Keep your lifting leg straight throughout the exercise. • Hold the top end of the bar so it does not roll off your ankle. • Keep your lifting leg close to your body.

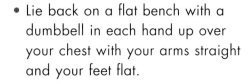

#4 DUMBBELL FLY

- Lie back on a flat bench with a dumbbell in each hand up over your chest with your arms straight and your feet flat.

- Lower the dumbbells to the sides of your body and down to shoulder level.

- Raise the dumbbells back up over your chest with straight arms.

HINTS

• You can increase the depth you take the dumbbells down as you get used to the exercise. • Lower and raise the dumbbells evenly to maintain balance. • Bend your elbows slightly to avoid stress on your shoulder joints as you lower the weights.

STRENGTH INTENSITY	TONE INTENSITY
3 sets	2 sets
12 reps	15 reps
45 seconds rest between sets	30 seconds rest between sets

#5 DUMBBELL UPRIGHT ROW

- Stand upright holding one dumbbell in each hand in front at your thighs with your arms straight and palms facing back.

- Lift the dumbbells straight up to just below your chin, keeping your elbows higher than your hands.

- Keep the dumbbells close to your body throughout the exercise.

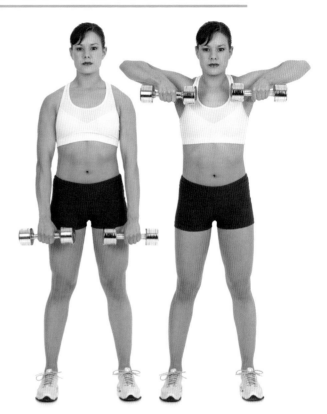

HINTS

• Always lift your elbows higher than your shoulders at the top of the exercise. • Do not turn your wrists. • Keep the dumbbells level throughout the exercise, and bring them close together at the top without banging them.

STRENGTH INTENSITY	TONE INTENSITY
3 sets	2 sets
12 reps	15 reps
45 seconds rest between sets	30 seconds rest between sets

#6 OBLIQUE CRUNCH

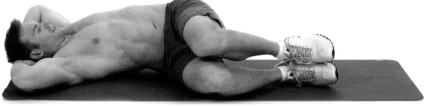

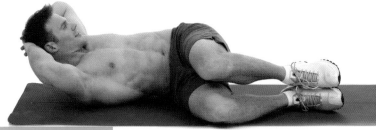

STRENGTH INTENSITY	TONE INTENSITY
3 sets	2 sets
12 reps	15 reps
45 seconds rest between sets	30 seconds rest between sets

- Lie on your back with your lower body twisted to one side, knees together and bent. Place your hands at the sides of your head.

- Lift your head and shoulders off the mat, keeping your lower body stable.

- Lower your head and shoulders and repeat. When you have completed the required number of reps, switch to the other side.

- Concentrate on contracting your abdominal muscles, and do not pull your head up with your hands.

HINTS

• Control the movement through your midsection and avoid jerky movements.
• Never use your hands to pull your head and neck up. • Lift only your head and shoulders off the floor, not your whole back. • Keep your legs together and turned to one side.

#7 FRONT BRIDGE

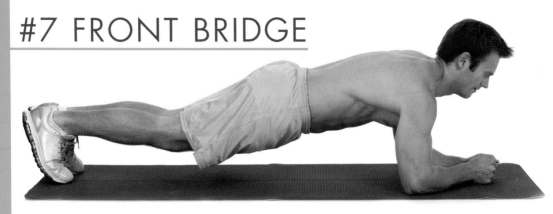

- Lie face down on the floor with your legs straight and arms tucked in by your sides.

- Lift your body off the floor, resting on your toes and forearms. Clasp your hands together to form an inverted V with your forearms.

- Keep your body in a straight line with a neutral or flat back.

- Hold this position for ten seconds, and then lower yourself back to the floor.

HINTS

• Start in a kneeling position with your elbows on the floor. Lift your hips and hold your torso in this position. • Keep both of your forearms on the floor with your elbows directly under your shoulders. • Start with your feet slightly apart.

STRENGTH INTENSITY	TONE INTENSITY
3 sets	2 sets
12 reps	15 reps
45 seconds rest between sets	30 seconds rest between sets

#8 JACKKNIFE

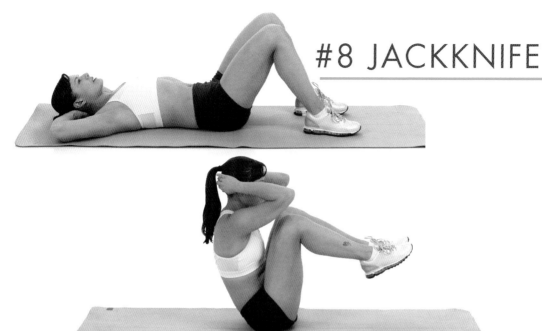

STRENGTH INTENSITY	TONE INTENSITY
3 sets	2 sets
12 reps	15 reps
45 seconds rest between sets	30 seconds rest between sets

- Lie on your back with your knees bent and feet flat. Place your hands at the sides of your head.

- Lift your head, shoulders, and back off the floor while bringing your knees in to your chest. Aim to get your elbows to meet your knees in the middle.

- Lower both your upper body and legs back to the floor.

HINT

• Use your abdominal muscles to control the movement through your midsection and avoid jerky movements. • Never use your hands to pull your head and neck up. • Think of folding up like a jackknife, as you lift your elbows to touch your knees.

#9 HAMSTRING STRETCH 4

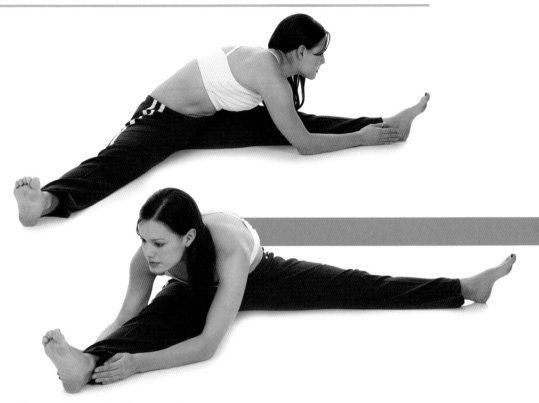

- Sit upright on the floor with your legs straight out to the sides. Lean forward to one side, bringing your chest to your knee and your hands to your ankle.

- Repeat on the other side.

- Bend your knees slightly, if necessary.

STRENGTH INTENSITY	TONE INTENSITY
Hold for 10 seconds. Repeat 3 times on each leg.	Hold for 10 seconds. Repeat 3 times on each leg.

#10 BACK STRETCH 1

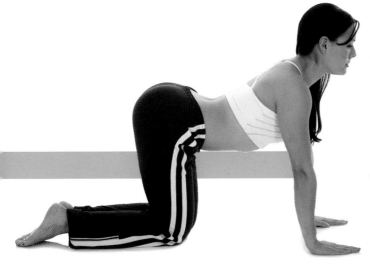

- Position yourself on all fours with your back slightly rounded and your head lifted and facing forward.

- Arch your back by pulling your abdominals in and up and raising your shoulders. Lower your head to look at the floor.

STRENGTH INTENSITY	TONE INTENSITY
Hold for 10 seconds. Repeat 3 times.	Hold for 10 seconds. Repeat 3 times.

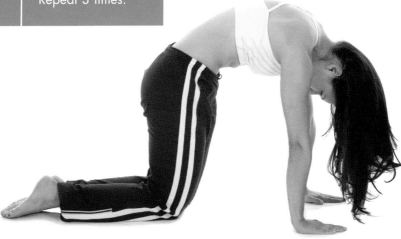

#11 GLUTE STRETCH 1

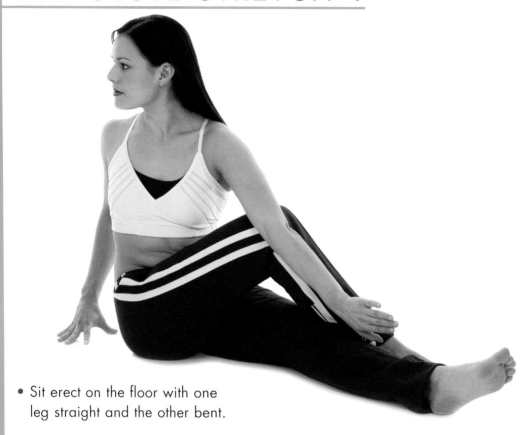

- Sit erect on the floor with one leg straight and the other bent.

- Cross the foot of the bent leg to the outside of the straight leg.

- With your arm straight, place your opposite elbow on the outside of your bent knee.

- Gently pull your knee across your body with your elbow as you look to the other side.

STRENGTH INTENSITY	TONE INTENSITY
Hold for 10 seconds. Repeat 3 times on each leg.	Hold for 10 seconds. Repeat 3 times on each leg.

#1 DUMBBELL STEP-UP

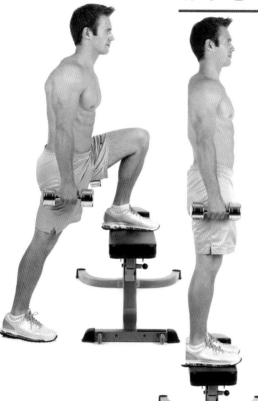

- Stand upright with one foot on a bench, holding a dumbbell at each side. Keep your head up and look straight forward.

- Step up onto the bench by pushing down on your top foot and leaning slightly forward.

- Step down off the bench onto the back foot, keeping the top foot on the bench, and repeat to complete your reps. Then switch to the other leg.

HINTS

- Maintain a neutral spine by keeping your head up and looking straight forward. • Place your body weight on the foot that is on the bench, not on the back foot. • Try not to push off using the back foot. Use the top foot to do the work. • Start with a low step and gradually increase the height.

STRENGTH INTENSITY	TONE INTENSITY
3 sets	2 sets
12 reps	15 reps
45 seconds rest between sets	30 seconds rest between sets

#2 MODIFIED SELF-ROW

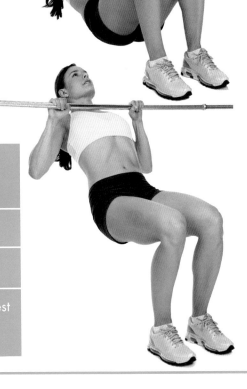

- Lie on the floor grasping a suspended straight bar with a wide grip, your arms straight, feet flat, and knees bent.

- Pull your body straight up to the bar to touch it with your chest. Keep your knees bent.

- Lower your body back toward the floor.

STRENGTH INTENSITY	TONE INTENSITY
3 sets	2 sets
12 reps	15 reps
45 seconds rest between sets	30 seconds rest between sets

HINTS

• Be sure that the bar is secure and can hold your weight. • Start with an underhanded grip until you are comfortable with an overhanded grip. • Just touch the bar with your mid-chest; do not touch the bar with your neck.

#3 GLUTE KICKBACK

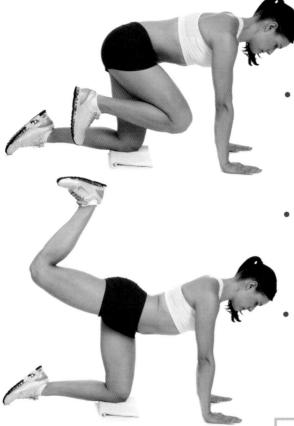

- Begin with both your knees and hands on the floor and your head in line with your spine. Look down at the floor.

- Bring one knee toward your chest, and then kick your leg back, lifting your foot up behind with your knee bent.

- Slowly lower your leg and repeat all reps on one leg before switching to the other side.

STRENGTH INTENSITY	TONE INTENSITY
3 sets	2 sets
12 reps	15 reps
45 seconds rest between sets	30 seconds rest between sets

HINTS

• Use smooth, controlled movements. Avoid jerky hip kicks that might force your lower back into hyperextension. • Modify the range of motion to begin and increase it as you get comfortable with the exercise.

#4 BARBELL BENCH PRESS

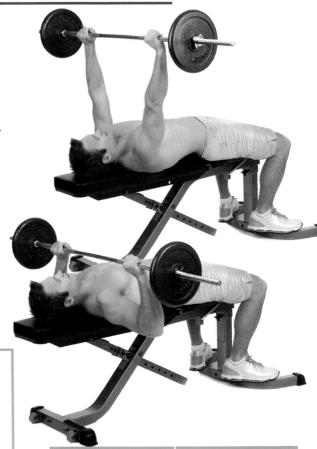

- Lie on a flat bench holding a large barbell straight up over your chest with your arms extended. Keep your hands shoulder-width apart. Place your feet flat on the floor.

- Lower the barbell down to the level of your mid-chest.

- Press the barbell back up to a straight-arm position.

HINTS

• Lower the barbell to your upper chest, not your neck. • Use an even grip so you are centered under the bar. • Do not bounce the bar off your chest; instead, barely touch it before pressing it back up.

STRENGTH INTENSITY	TONE INTENSITY
3 sets	2 sets
12 reps	15 reps
45 seconds rest between sets	30 seconds rest between sets

#5 DUMBBELL LATERAL RAISE

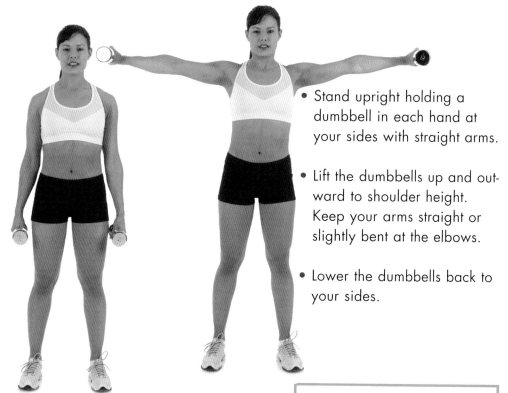

- Stand upright holding a dumbbell in each hand at your sides with straight arms.

- Lift the dumbbells up and outward to shoulder height. Keep your arms straight or slightly bent at the elbows.

- Lower the dumbbells back to your sides.

STRENGTH INTENSITY	TONE INTENSITY
3 sets	2 sets
12 reps	15 reps
45 seconds rest between sets	30 seconds rest between sets

HINTS

• Keep your back upright by contracting your core muscles as you raise the dumbbells. • Avoid jerky movements. • Bend your elbows slightly to avoid too much stress on your shoulder joints. • Start with your feet about shoulder-width apart. To challenge your stability, bring your feet closer together.

#6 REVERSE CRUNCH

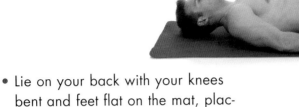

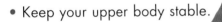

- Lie on your back with your knees bent and feet flat on the mat, placing your hands at your sides.

- Bring your knees up to your chest with your legs bent, slightly rounding your lower back at the top position.

- Keep your upper body stable.

- Slowly lower your legs with your knees still bent to tap your heels on the floor.

HINTS

• Keep your upper back and shoulders on the mat. • Do not change your leg position. Keep your knees bent at the same angle throughout the exercise.
• Go through the full range of motion, tapping your heels on the floor each time.

STRENGTH INTENSITY	TONE INTENSITY
3 sets	2 sets
12 reps	15 reps
45 seconds rest between sets	30 seconds rest between sets

#7 QUAD FLYER

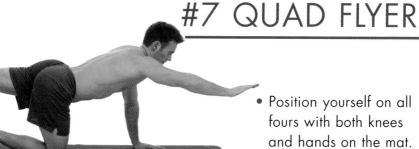

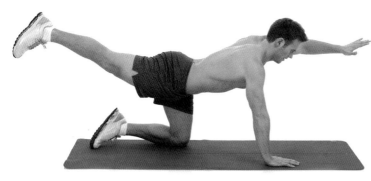

- Position yourself on all fours with both knees and hands on the mat.

- Lift one arm and the opposite leg straight up to shoulder height.

- Slowly lower your arm and leg and repeat the lift with the other arm and leg.

- Take your time and maintain your balance.

STRENGTH INTENSITY	TONE INTENSITY
3 sets	2 sets
12 reps	15 reps
45 seconds rest between sets	30 seconds rest between sets

HINTS

• Control the lifts with your core muscles. Avoid throwing your arms and legs up in the air. • Lift both your legs and arms up to the same height, and keep your head steady. • Do not raise your head as you lift your arm and leg; keep it in line with your spine.

#8 FLUTTER KICKS

- Lie flat on your back with your legs straight and your arms by your sides.

- Lift one leg straight about 12 inches, then the other to about 12 inches above that.

- Continue to raise your legs, one at a time, as if you were taking mini-steps.

- Move your legs up and then back down in sequence of steps one at a time.

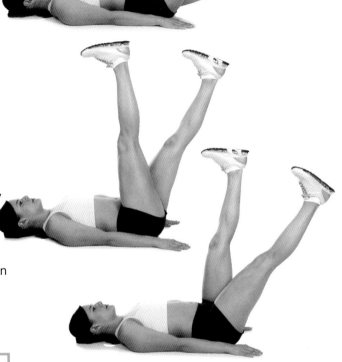

HINTS

• Keep your legs straight. • Use small movements, alternating legs, on both the way up and down. • Keep your hips on the floor.

STRENGTH INTENSITY	TONE INTENSITY
3 sets	2 sets
12 reps	15 reps
45 seconds rest between sets	30 seconds rest between sets

#9 HIP FLEXOR STRETCH 2

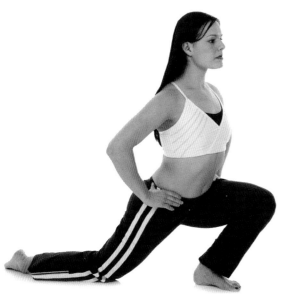

- With one knee on the floor, step slightly forward with the other leg into a lunge.

- Lean into your front foot, pushing your back hip toward the floor.

- Raise your back heel to your buttocks, holding it at the ankle.

- Gently pull your foot closer to your buttocks to feel a greater stretch.

- Brace yourself with your hand on the forward leg.

STRENGTH INTENSITY	TONE INTENSITY
Hold for 10 seconds. Repeat 3 times on each leg.	Hold for 10 seconds. Repeat 3 times on each leg.

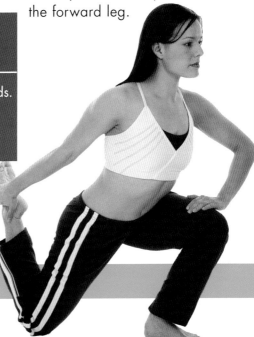

#10 PECTORAL STRETCH WITH SWISS BALL

- Lie with your mid-back on the Swiss ball and your hands at the sides of your head.

- Roll back slightly on the ball, opening your chest and extending your arms overhead toward the floor.

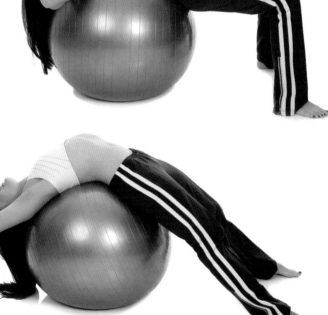

STRENGTH INTENSITY	TONE INTENSITY
Hold for 10 seconds. Repeat 3 times.	Hold for 10 seconds. Repeat 3 times.

#11 HAMSTRING STRETCH 2

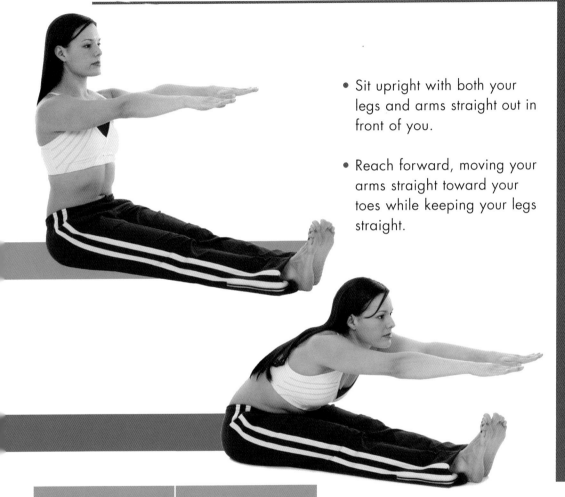

- Sit upright with both your legs and arms straight out in front of you.

- Reach forward, moving your arms straight toward your toes while keeping your legs straight.

STRENGTH INTENSITY	TONE INTENSITY
Hold for 10 seconds. Repeat 3 times.	Hold for 10 seconds. Repeat 3 times.

#1 DUMBBELL REVERSE LUNGE

- Stand upright holding a dumbbell in each hand by your sides, head up and looking straight forward.

- Take a step backward, and drop your back knee toward the floor, bending at the hip and knee.

- Lean slightly forward, keeping all your weight on your front foot.

- Push off your front foot to return to the starting position. Repeat on the other side.

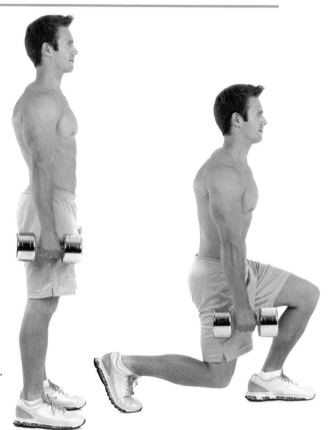

HINTS

• Keep your body weight over your front foot. • Lean forward slightly as if you were bending down to put something on the floor in front of you. Maintain a flat or neutral spine. • Keep your head up and back flat throughout the exercise.

STRENGTH INTENSITY	TONE INTENSITY
3 sets	2 sets
12 reps	15 reps
45 seconds rest between sets	30 seconds rest between sets

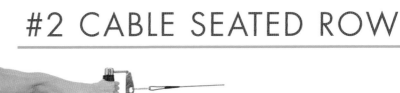

#2 CABLE SEATED ROW

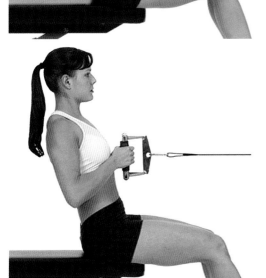

- Sit upright on a bench, holding the cable handle with your arms straight out in front. Keep your back flat.

- Pull the cable handle straight in to your chest, bending at your elbows.

- Slowly, extend your arms to return the handle to the starting position.

HINTS

• As you pull the handle in, expand your chest slightly and pull your shoulder blades together. • Keep your back upright and steady as you pull the handle in and out. • Keep your head up, looking straight forward, and do not lift your shoulders. • Your elbows should move backward close to your sides—not outward.

STRENGTH INTENSITY	TONE INTENSITY
3 sets	2 sets
12 reps	15 reps
45 seconds rest between sets	30 seconds rest between sets

#3 STRAIGHT BAR HIP ADDUCTION

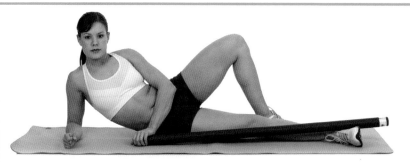

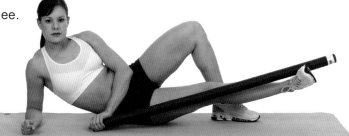

- Lie on your side with your bottom leg straight and a straight bar resting across that ankle. Bend your other knee.

- Raise your leg and the bar straight up. Slowly lower your leg and the bar back to the floor.

- Perform all the specified reps on one side, and then switch legs.

HINTS

• Keep your lifting leg straight throughout the exercise. • Hold the top end of the bar so it does not roll off your ankle. • Keep your lifting leg close to your body.

STRENGTH INTENSITY	TONE INTENSITY
3 sets	2 sets
12 reps	15 reps
45 seconds rest between sets	30 seconds rest between sets

#4 DUMBBELL PULLOVER

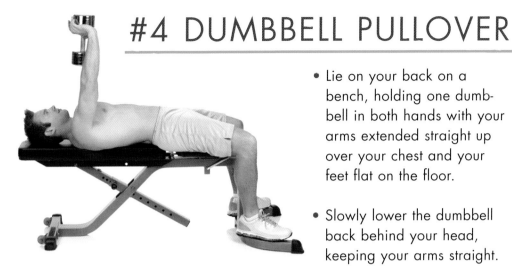

- Lie on your back on a bench, holding one dumb-bell in both hands with your arms extended straight up over your chest and your feet flat on the floor.

- Slowly lower the dumbbell back behind your head, keeping your arms straight.

- Lower until your hands are in line with your shoulders.

- Lift the dumbbell back up, returning to the starting position.

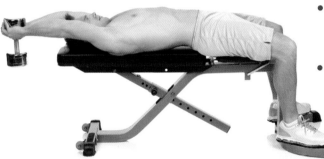

STRENGTH INTENSITY	TONE INTENSITY
3 sets	2 sets
12 reps	15 reps
45 seconds rest between sets	30 seconds rest between sets

HINTS

• Bend your elbows slightly as you lower your arms. • Lower the dumbbell farther behind your head when you feel comfortable with the exercise. • Keep your feet flat on the floor to maintain balance.

#5 PRONE DUMBBELL BACK DELT ROW

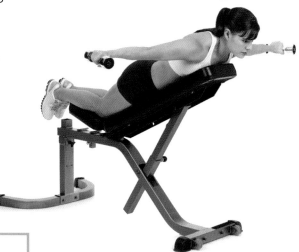

- Position yourself face down on an incline bench with a dumbbell in each hand hanging at your sides. Your arms should be straight and your palms facing in.

- Lift the dumbbells up and out to the side to shoulder height, keeping your arms straight.

- Lower the dumbbells back to a vertical position.

- Bend your elbows slightly, if necessary.

HINTS

• Move smoothly and don't bounce at the top of the position. • Draw your arms up and out to the side, pulling your shoulder blades together. • Look at the floor to keep your head in line with your spine. • Do not lift your head as you lift the dumbbell.

STRENGTH INTENSITY	TONE INTENSITY
3 sets	2 sets
12 reps	15 reps
45 seconds rest between sets	30 seconds rest between sets

#6 TWISTING CRUNCH

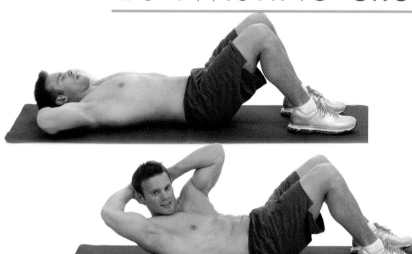

STRENGTH INTENSITY	TONE INTENSITY
3 sets	2 sets
12 reps	15 reps
45 seconds rest between sets	30 seconds rest between sets

- Lie on your back with your knees raised and bent and your feet flat on the mat, placing your hands at the sides of your head.

- Lift your head and shoulders off the floor and twist your torso to one side as if you were trying to touch the opposite knee with your elbow.

- Lower your head and shoulders, then repeat, twisting to the other side.

- Keep your feet flat on the floor.

HINTS

• Use your core muscles to control the twist through your midsection. Move smoothly.
• Don't use your hands to pull your head and neck up. • Lift only your head and shoulders, not your whole back. • Start with your feet about shoulder-width apart.

#7 SWISS BALL T

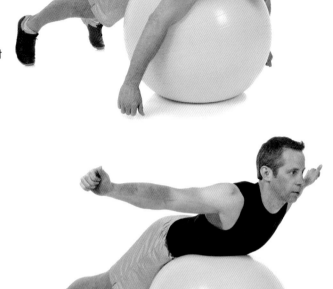

- Lie face down over a Swiss ball resting on your mid-chest with your toes touching the floor and your arms hanging forward over the ball.

- Lift your upper body off the ball, bringing your arms up straight out to the sides to form a T.

- Hold this position for ten seconds. Lower your body back to the ball.

HINTS

- Lift yourself only to the point where your chest is off the ball.
- Keep your upper body straight at the top of the exercise. • Do not over-arch your lower back. • Push your toes into the floor to help keep you stable.

STRENGTH INTENSITY	TONE INTENSITY
3 sets	2 sets
12 reps	15 reps
45 seconds rest between sets	30 seconds rest between sets

#8 OBLIQUE BRIDGE

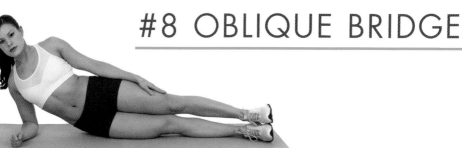

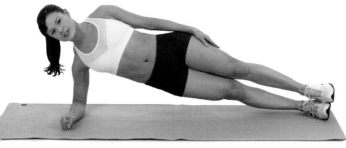

- Lie on one side, propped up on one forearm with your legs straight out, one on top of the another. Position your other arm along the top of your body.

- Lift your body up off the floor, resting on your forearm and bottom foot.

- Hold the position for ten seconds, and then lower yourself back to the floor.

- Repeat to complete your reps and then switch to the other side.

STRENGTH INTENSITY	TONE INTENSITY
3 sets	2 sets
12 reps	15 reps
45 seconds rest between sets	30 seconds rest between sets

HINTS

- Try to keep your body in a straight line with your elbow directly under your shoulder.
- Keep one foot on top of the other, if possible. For better balance, you can put both feet on the floor. • Position your top hand on the floor if you need help with balance.

#9 HAMSTRING STRETCH 1

- Lie on your back with both legs straight out ahead on the floor.

- Lift one leg straight up, grasp it behind your calf or ankle, and gently pull it toward your head.

- You may bend your knee slighly.

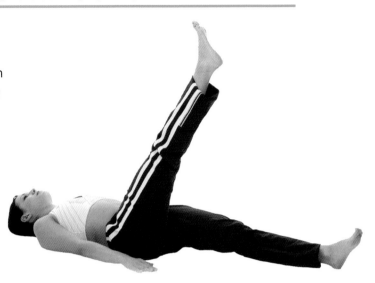

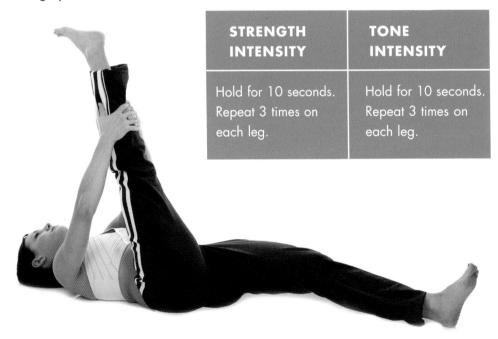

STRENGTH INTENSITY	TONE INTENSITY
Hold for 10 seconds. Repeat 3 times on each leg.	Hold for 10 seconds. Repeat 3 times on each leg.

#10 BACK STRETCH 2

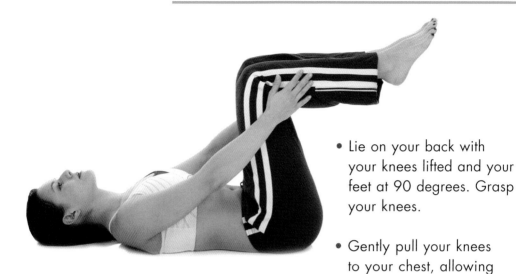

- Lie on your back with your knees lifted and your feet at 90 degrees. Grasp your knees.

- Gently pull your knees to your chest, allowing your lower back to round slightly.

STRENGTH INTENSITY	TONE INTENSITY
Hold for 10 seconds. Repeat 3 times.	Hold for 10 seconds. Repeat 3 times.

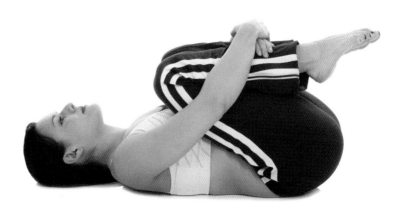

#11 GLUTE STRETCH 2

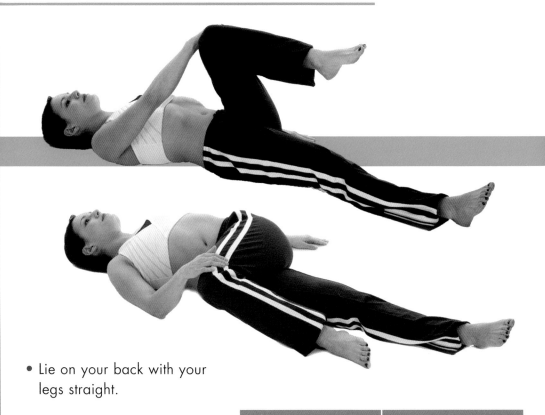

- Lie on your back with your legs straight.

- Bring one leg up and across your body, bending it at the knee.

- Use your opposite hand to pull your knee across and down toward the floor.

STRENGTH INTENSITY	TONE INTENSITY
Hold for 10 seconds. Repeat 3 times on each leg.	Hold for 10 seconds. Repeat 3 times on each leg.

#1 DUMBBELL SQUAT

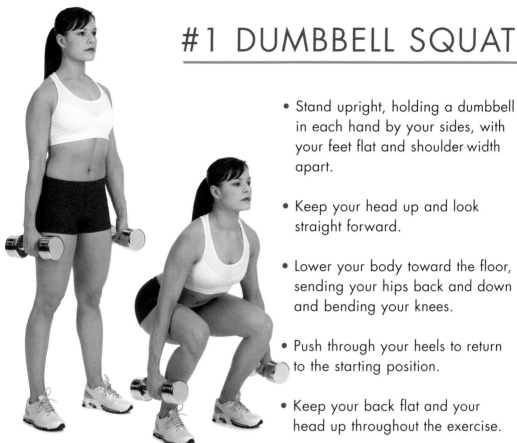

- Stand upright, holding a dumbbell in each hand by your sides, with your feet flat and shoulder-width apart.

- Keep your head up and look straight forward.

- Lower your body toward the floor, sending your hips back and down and bending your knees.

- Push through your heels to return to the starting position.

- Keep your back flat and your head up throughout the exercise.

STRENGTH INTENSITY	TONE INTENSITY
3 sets	3 sets
10 reps	12 reps
45 seconds rest between sets	30 seconds rest between sets

HINTS

• Back position is very important in squatting exercises. Always maintain a neutral position and do not round your lower back or over-arch it. • Keep your head up, looking straight forward, and keep your shoulders back to help prevent rounding your upper back. • Keep the dumbbells at the sides of your legs, not in front.

#2 CABLE STANDING ROW

- Stand upright, holding the cable handle with your arms straight out in front, your knees slightly bent, and your back flat.

- Pull the cable handle straight in to your chest.

- Keep upright and steady.

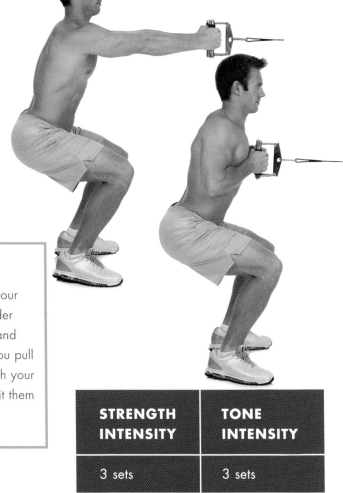

HINTS

• At the end of the exercise, lift your chest slightly and pull your shoulder blades together. • Keep upright and do not sway back and forth as you pull the handle in and out. • Start with your feet about hip-width apart, or split them front to back for more stability.

STRENGTH INTENSITY	TONE INTENSITY
3 sets	3 sets
10 reps	12 reps
45 seconds rest between sets	30 seconds rest between sets

#3 STIFF-LEG DUMBBELL DEADLIFT

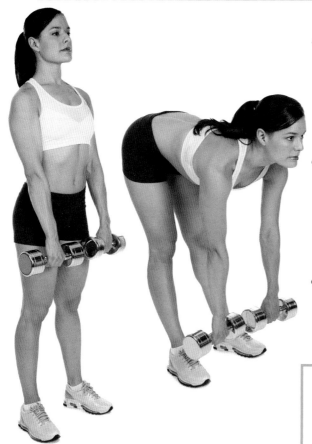

- Stand upright, holding a dumbbell in each hand at your thighs, with your arms straight and your feet hip-width apart.

- Lower the dumbbells to below your knees, shifting your hips back and keeping your legs straight and your back flat.

- Return to the upright starting position.

HINTS

- Start gradually and increase your range of motion as you become more comfortable with the exercise. • Do not round your lower back. • Stop at a point where you are no longer shifting your hips backward.
- Do not bounce in the bent position.

STRENGTH INTENSITY	TONE INTENSITY
3 sets	3 sets
10 reps	12 reps
45 seconds rest between sets	30 seconds rest between sets

#4 RAISED-FEET BENCH DIP

- Position yourself with your palms behind you on a bench and your heels in front on another bench. Keep your legs and arms straight.

- Bending your elbows, lower your body toward the floor.

- Push up through your palms to return to the starting position.

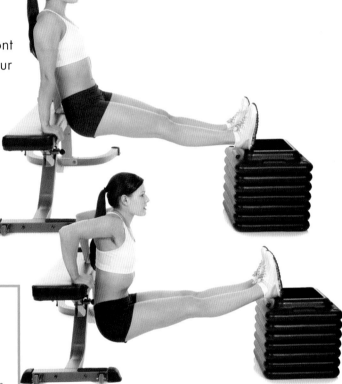

HINTS

- Start by sitting on the bench with your feet on the floor. Place your feet on the other bench, then position your hands on the edge of the bench. • Keep your head up and look straight forward to maintain a neutral back position.
- When you feel comfortable with the exercise, try to lower yourself a bit farther.

STRENGTH INTENSITY	TONE INTENSITY
3 sets	3 sets
10 reps	12 reps
45 seconds rest between sets	30 seconds rest between sets

#5 BARBELL OVERHEAD PRESS

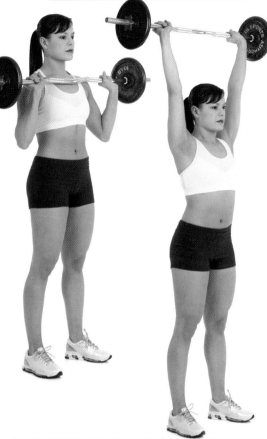

- Stand upright holding a large barbell at shoulder height in front with your hands shoulder-width apart, your elbows bent, and your palms facing forward.

- Press the barbell overhead, extending your arms fully.

- Lower the barbell by bending your elbows to the starting position with the barbell at your shoulder level.

HINTS

• Keep your back straight by contracting your core muscles as you push the barbell overhead. • Complete the full range of motion from shoulder level to arms fully extended overhead and back again. • Start with your feet about shoulder-width apart and your hands evenly spaced on the barbell. • To challenge your stability, bring your feet closer together.

STRENGTH INTENSITY	TONE INTENSITY
3 sets	3 sets
10 reps	12 reps
45 seconds rest between sets	30 seconds rest between sets

#6 SWISS BALL REVERSE EXTENSION

- Lie face down on a Swiss ball, resting on your lower abdomen, with your hands and feet touching the floor.

- Lift both legs straight up until your ankles, hips, and shoulders are in line.

- Slowly lower your body back to the floor. Do not bounce on the ball.

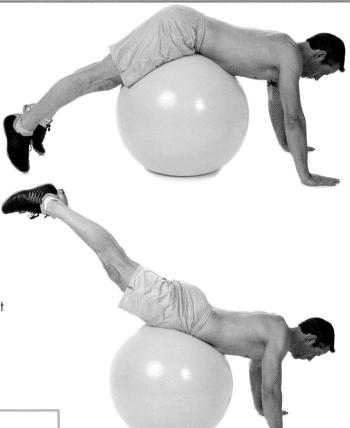

HINTS

- Move smoothly and with control. Don't throw your legs up in the air.
- Do not over-arch your lower back. Come up just to the point where your feet are in line with your hips.
- Keep your hands and feet wide apart to help maintain balance.

STRENGTH INTENSITY	TONE INTENSITY
3 sets	3 sets
10 reps	12 reps
45 seconds rest between sets	30 seconds rest between sets

#7 ALTERNATING BRIDGE

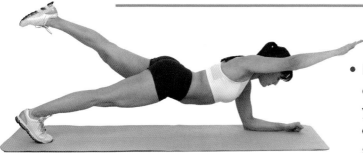

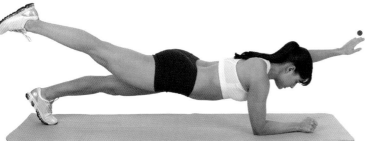

- Position yourself face down on a mat with your legs straight and arms tucked in by your sides.

- Lift your body off the mat, resting on your toes and forearms, then lift one arm and the opposite leg about 18 inches off the floor.

- Hold for ten seconds, then lower yourself back to the floor and repeat with the other arm and opposite leg.

- Hold your body in a straight line, and keep your back in a neutral position throughout.

STRENGTH INTENSITY	TONE INTENSITY
3 sets	3 sets
10 reps	12 reps
45 seconds rest between sets	30 seconds rest between sets

HINTS

- Use your core muscles to control the movements, and don't thrust yourself up off the floor.
- Lift both legs and arms up to the same height, keeping your head steady. • Do not lift your head as you raise your arm and leg; keep it in line with your spine.

#8 HIGH-LOW CABLE CHOP

- Stand upright with your upper torso facing one side. Grasp a cable handle in both hands with straight arms, twisting over one shoulder.

- Pull the cable handle down below your shoulder and across your body to the outside of your opposite hip.

- Repeat on the other side.

- Concentrate on moving your hips and shoulders, not your arms.

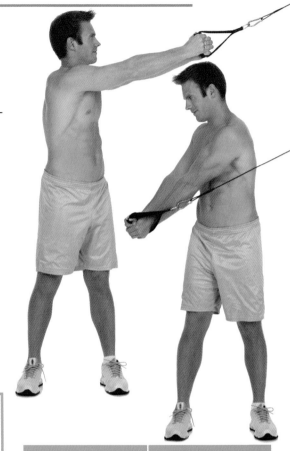

HINTS

- As if chopping a tree, pull the cable down from over your shoulder and across your body to the opposite side. • Move smoothly and avoid jerky movements.
- Rotate through your hips and shoulders, keeping your arms straight. • Shift your feet, if necessary.

STRENGTH INTENSITY	TONE INTENSITY
3 sets	3 sets
10 reps	12 reps
45 seconds rest between sets	30 seconds rest between sets

#9 UPWARD DOG

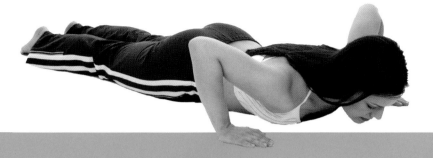

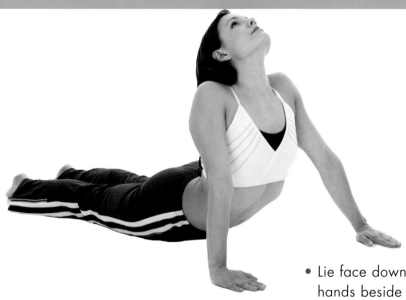

STRENGTH INTENSITY	TONE INTENSITY
Hold for 10 seconds. Repeat 3 times.	Hold for 10 seconds. Repeat 3 times.

- Lie face down with your hands beside your shoulders and your elbows bent, chin touching the floor.

- Push up your upper body, arching your back while keeping your hips and legs on the floor.

#10 HAMSTRING STRETCH 2

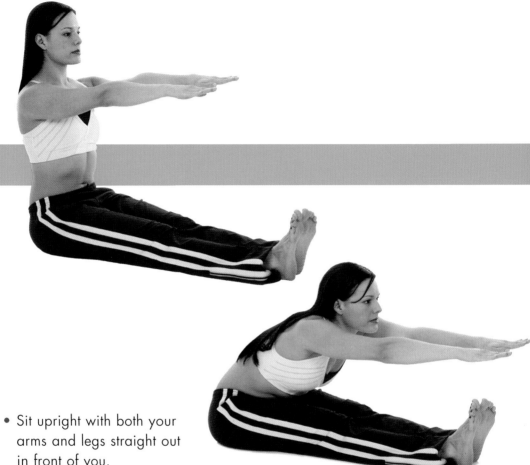

- Sit upright with both your arms and legs straight out in front of you.

- Lean forward with straight arms, reaching toward your toes and keeping your legs straight.

STRENGTH INTENSITY	TONE INTENSITY
Hold for 10 seconds. Repeat 3 times.	Hold for 10 seconds. Repeat 3 times.

#11 HIP FLEXOR STRETCH 1

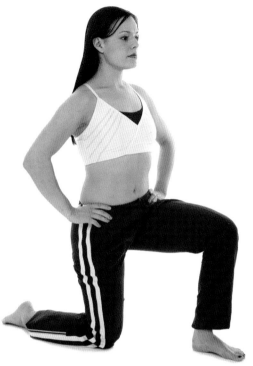

- With one knee on the floor, position the other leg slightly forward.

- Shift your weight onto your front foot, pushing your back hip toward the floor.

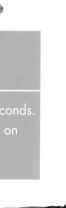

STRENGTH INTENSITY	TONE INTENSITY
Hold for 10 seconds. Repeat 3 times on each leg.	Hold for 10 seconds. Repeat 3 times on each leg.

#1 BARBELL BACK SQUAT

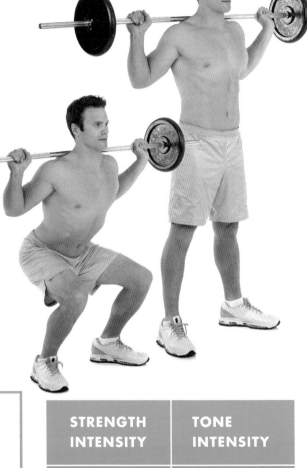

- Stand upright with a large barbell behind your shoulders and your feet flat and shoulder-width apart.

- Keep your head up, looking straight forward.

- Lower your body toward the floor, bending your knees to send your hips back and down.

- Push through your heels to return to the starting position.

- Keep your back flat and head up throughout the exercise.

HINTS

• Back position is very important in squatting exercises. Always maintain a neutral position; do not round the lower back or over-arch it. • Keep your head up, looking straight forward, with your shoulders back. • Position the barbell at the back of your shoulders, not across the back of your neck. • Maintain a wide grip on the barbell to keep it from rolling.

STRENGTH INTENSITY	TONE INTENSITY
3 sets	3 sets
10 reps	12 reps
45 seconds rest between sets	30 seconds rest between sets

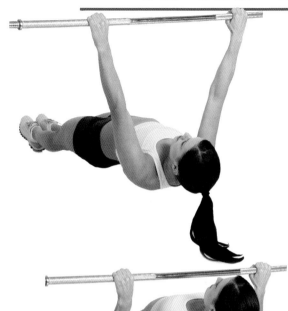

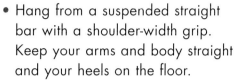

- Hang from a suspended straight bar with a shoulder-width grip. Keep your arms and body straight and your heels on the floor.

- Pull your body straight up to the bar to touch it with your chest.

- Lower your body back to a straight-arm position.

HINTS

• Be sure that the bar is secure and can hold your weight. • Start with an under-handed grip, then switch to an over-handed grip when you are comfortable with the exercise. • Pull yourself up so your chest, not your neck, just touches the bar.

STRENGTH INTENSITY	TONE INTENSITY
3 sets	3 sets
10 reps	12 reps
45 seconds rest between sets	30 seconds rest between sets

#3 DUMBBELL SIDE LUNGE

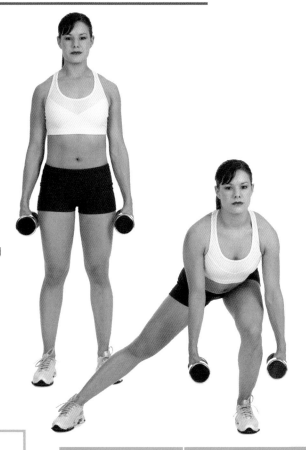

- Stand upright holding a dumbbell in each hand by your sides. Keep your head up, looking straight forward.

- Step to one side, lowering your body into a half squat and leaning slightly forward with your weight on your outside leg. Keep your trailing leg straight.

- Push off your outside foot to return to the starting position.

- Repeat the exercise on the other leg.

HINTS

• Maintain a neutral back position; do not round your lower back or over-arch it. • Keep your head up, looking straight forward, with your shoulders back. • Place your body weight over your outside foot to help maintain balance and to push off with. • Keep the other leg straight throughout.

STRENGTH INTENSITY	TONE INTENSITY
3 sets	3 sets
10 reps	12 reps
45 seconds rest between sets	30 seconds rest between sets

#4 BARBELL BENCH PRESS

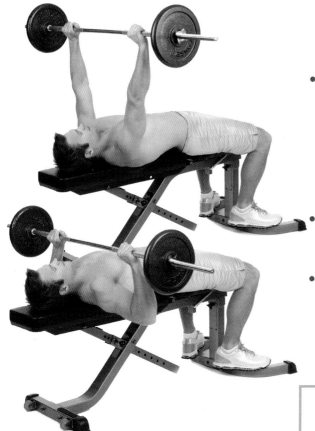

- Lie on a flat bench holding a large barbell in both hands with your arms extended straight up over your chest, keeping your hands shoulder-width apart.

- Lower the barbell down to mid-chest level.

- Press the barbell back up to a straight-arm position.

STRENGTH INTENSITY	TONE INTENSITY
3 sets	3 sets
10 reps	12 reps
45 seconds rest between sets	30 seconds rest between sets

HINTS

• Lower the barbell just to your upper chest level, not to your neck. • Take an even grip so you are centered under the barbell. • Do not bounce the barbell off your chest. Instead, barely touch your chest before pressing the barbell back up.

#5 DUMBBELL FRONT RAISE

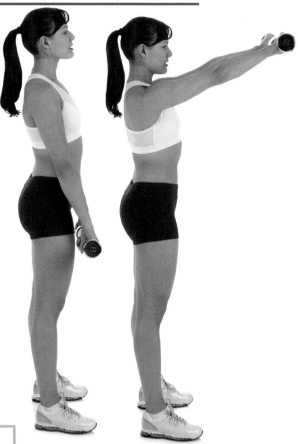

- Stand upright holding a dumbbell in each hand in front of your hips. Position your arms straight with your palms facing back.

- Lift the dumbbells to shoulder height in front. Keep your arms straight.

- Lower the dumbbells to the starting position and repeat.

HINTS

- Keep your back upright by contracting your core muscles as you lift the dumbbells. • Avoid jerky movements.
- Bend your elbows slightly to avoid stress on your shoulder joints. • Start with your feet about hip-width apart.

STRENGTH INTENSITY	TONE INTENSITY
3 sets	3 sets
10 reps	12 reps
45 seconds rest between sets	30 seconds rest between sets

#6 MEDICINE BALL TWIST

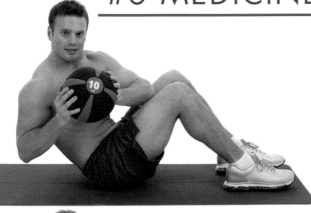

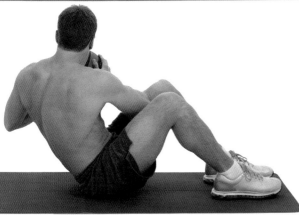

- Start in a sit-up position with your feet flat and your knees bent, holding a medicine ball with both hands.

- Twist your torso to one side, lowering the medicine ball toward the floor.

- Twist back to the other side.

STRENGTH INTENSITY	TONE INTENSITY
3 sets	3 sets
10 reps	12 reps
45 seconds rest between sets	30 seconds rest between sets

HINTS

- Keep your feet flat on the floor throughout the exercise. • Twist through your entire midsection. Do not just move your arms.
- Turn both your head and shoulders to the sides for each rep.

#7 SWISS BALL ELBOW BRIDGE

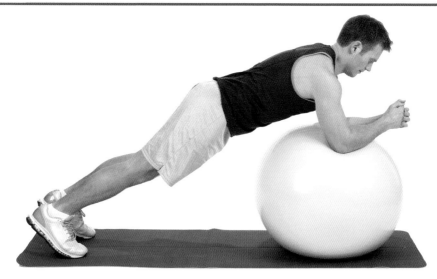

- Position yourself with your forearms on a Swiss ball and your legs extended, with both feet on the floor.

- Keep the ball directly under your chest and your body straight.

- Hold this position for ten seconds and then lower your body down to lie on the ball.

STRENGTH INTENSITY	TONE INTENSITY
3 sets	3 sets
10 reps	12 reps
45 seconds rest between sets	30 seconds rest between sets

HINTS

- Start in a kneeling position with your elbows on the ball. Raise your hips to get in position and hold it throughout the movement. • Keep your forearms on top of the ball.
- Start with your feet hip-width apart.

#8 SIDE BRIDGE WITH ABDUCTION

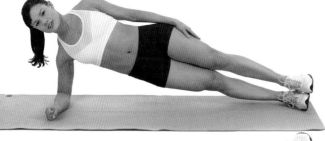

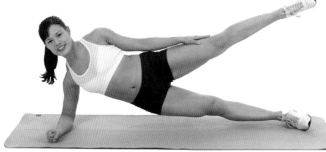

- Start by lying on one side propped up on one elbow with your legs straight out, one on top of the other.

- Lift your body off the floor, resting on your forearm and bottom foot.

- Lift your top leg up, keeping it straight, with the rest of your body in a straight line and your elbow directly under your shoulder.

- Hold for ten seconds, then lower yourself back to the floor.

- Complete your reps and then switch to the other side.

STRENGTH INTENSITY	TONE INTENSITY
3 sets	3 sets
10 reps	12 reps
45 seconds rest between sets	30 seconds rest between sets

HINTS

• Keep your body in a straight line with your elbow directly under your shoulder. • Keep one foot on top of the other, if possible. • Beginning with both feet on the floor helps you balance. • Keep the raised leg in line with the other leg as you lift it. • Placing your top hand on the floor also helps maintain balance.

#9 BACK STRETCH 3

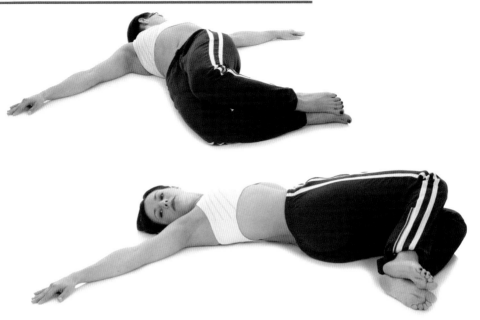

- Lie flat on your back with your knees bent and feet together. Extend your arms straight out to the sides at shoulder height.

- Lower your knees to touch the floor on one side as you turn your head to the other side.

- Repeat, twisting to the opposite side, switching both your legs and head position.

STRENGTH INTENSITY	TONE INTENSITY
Hold for 10 seconds. Repeat 3 times on each side.	Hold for 10 seconds. Repeat 3 times on each side.

#10 HAMSTRING STRETCH 1

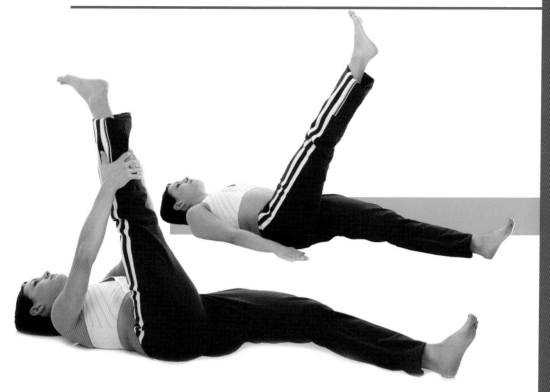

STRENGTH INTENSITY	TONE INTENSITY
Hold for 10 seconds. Repeat 3 times on each leg.	Hold for 10 seconds. Repeat 3 times on each leg.

- Lie on your back with both legs straight out on the floor. Raise one leg straight up.

- Grasp behind the calf or ankle of the lifted leg and gently pull it toward your head.

- Bend your knees slightly, if necessary.

#11 QUADRICEPS STRETCH 1

- Stand upright on one leg, bending the other leg at the knee and pulling the heel back to your buttocks. Grasp your ankle with one hand and gently pull your foot closer to get a deeper stretch.

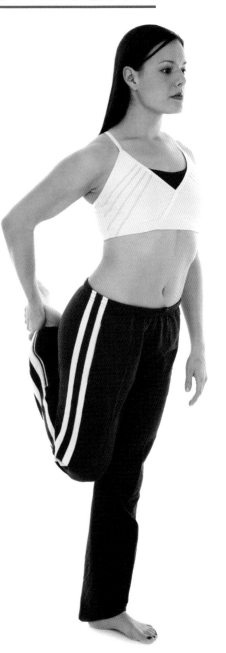

STRENGTH INTENSITY	TONE INTENSITY
Hold for 10 seconds. Repeat 3 times on each leg.	Hold for 10 seconds. Repeat 3 times on each leg.

#1 BARBELL DEADLIFT

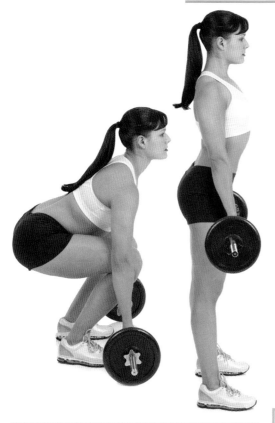

- Start in a squat position with your feet hip-width apart, your head up, and your hips low, grasping a barbell on the floor.

- Keep your head up and look straight forward.

- Stand up, lifting the barbell while keeping your arms straight and your back flat.

- Lower the barbell to the floor, sending your hips back and down and bending your knees.

STRENGTH INTENSITY	TONE INTENSITY
3 sets	3 sets
10 reps	12 reps
45 seconds rest between sets	30 seconds rest between sets

HINTS

• Keep your back in a neutral position. Do not round your lower back. • Hold your head up, looking straight forward, and keep your shoulders back. • Keep the barbell close to your body throughout the exercise. • Slowly lower the barbell back to the floor at the end of each rep.

#2 BILATERAL DUMBBELL BENT-OVER ROW

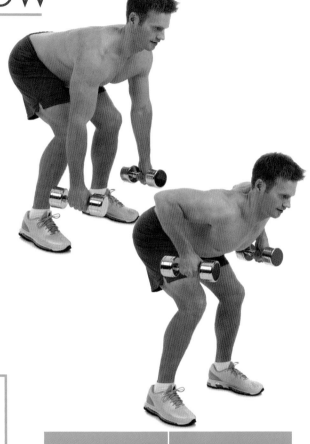

- Hold a dumbbell in each hand with your arms straight and your palms facing in.

- Bend forward at your waist with your knees slightly bent while keeping your back flat.

- Lift the dumbbells along the sides of your chest, with your elbows up and back.

- Lower the dumbbells back to a straight-arm position, keeping your back flat.

HINTS

- Look down as you perform the movement to maintain a neutral spine.
- Do not raise your head as you lift the dumbbells. • As you lift the dumbbells, draw your elbows up close by your sides, not outward. • Lift the dumbbells until your elbows are above your shoulders.

STRENGTH INTENSITY	TONE INTENSITY
3 sets	3 sets
10 reps	12 reps
45 seconds rest between sets	30 seconds rest between sets

#3 DUMBBELL STEP-UP

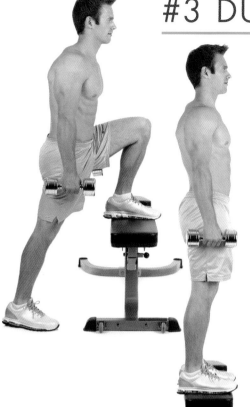

- Stand upright, holding a dumbbell in each hand by your sides.

- Place one foot on a chair or bench and keep the other flat on the floor. Lean forward, shifting your body weight onto the foot on the chair.

- Push down onto the front foot on the chair and step up with the other foot.

- Step down off the chair onto the back foot.

- Once you have completed your reps, repeat on the other leg.

HINTS

• Keep your head up and look straight forward to keep your spine neutral. • Place your body weight on the foot that is on the chair, not on the back foot. • Don't push off with your back foot. Use your top foot to do the work. • Start with a low step and gradually increase the height.

STRENGTH INTENSITY	TONE INTENSITY
3 sets	3 sets
10 reps	12 reps
45 seconds rest between sets	30 seconds rest between sets

#4 BARBELL PULLOVER

- Lie on your back, grasping a large barbell with your arms extended straight over your chest.

- Slowly lower the barbell back behind your head, keeping your arms straight.

- Move the barbell down until your hands are in line with your shoulders.

- Lift the barbell back up over your chest, returning to the starting position.

HINTS

- Space your hands evenly on the barbell.
- Bend your elbows slightly as you lower the barbell. • Lower the barbell farther behind your head when you feel comfortable with the exercise. • Keep your feet flat on the floor or on a bench to maintain balance.

STRENGTH INTENSITY	TONE INTENSITY
3 sets	3 sets
10 reps	12 reps
45 seconds rest between sets	30 seconds rest between sets

#5 BARBELL UPRIGHT ROW

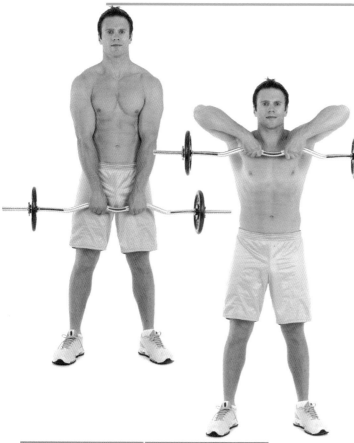

- Stand upright holding a barbell with your hands close together with an overhand grip and your arms straight with your palms facing back.

- Lift the barbell up to a point just below your chin, keeping your elbows above your hands.

STRENGTH INTENSITY	TONE INTENSITY
3 sets	3 sets
10 reps	12 reps
45 seconds rest between sets	30 seconds rest between sets

HINTS

• Grip the barbell with your hands close together near the middle of the bar. • Keep your spine upright and steady. • Hold your elbows higher than your shoulders when you have lifted the barbell. • Keep the barbell close to your body throughout the exercise.

#6 FLYER

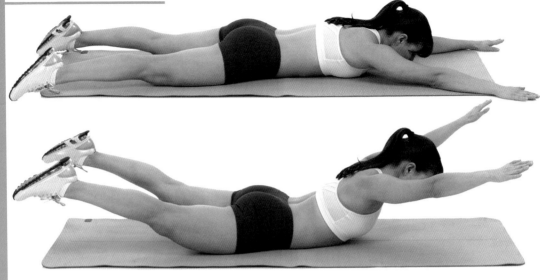

- Lie face down on a mat with your legs straight behind you and your arms stretched out in front.

- Lift your upper body and legs simultaneously to about 18 inches off the floor as if you were flying.

- Hold this position for ten seconds, then lower yourself back to the floor.

STRENGTH INTENSITY	TONE INTENSITY
3 sets	3 sets
10 reps	12 reps
45 seconds rest between sets	30 seconds rest between sets

HINTS

- Use your core muscles to control the lifts. Avoid throwing yourself up off the floor.
- Lift both your legs and arms to the same height, and keep your head steady throughout. • Do not over-extend your lower back.

#7 REVERSE HYPEREXTENSION

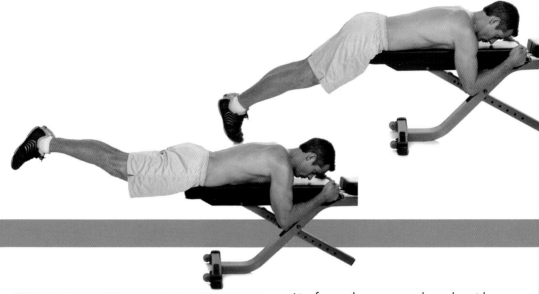

STRENGTH INTENSITY	TONE INTENSITY
3 sets	3 sets
10 reps	12 reps
45 seconds rest between sets	30 seconds rest between sets

- Lie face down on a bench with your lower body off the bench and your toes touching the floor.

- Lift your lower body until your whole body is in a straight line.

- Lower your legs to tap the floor.

- Hold on to the top of the bench for stability.

HINTS

• Move smoothly and do not throw your legs up in the air. • Never over-arch your lower back. • Lift your feet to the same height as your hips or just slightly higher. • Hold onto the bench and keep your feet wide to help maintain your balance.

#8 LOW-HIGH CABLE CHOP

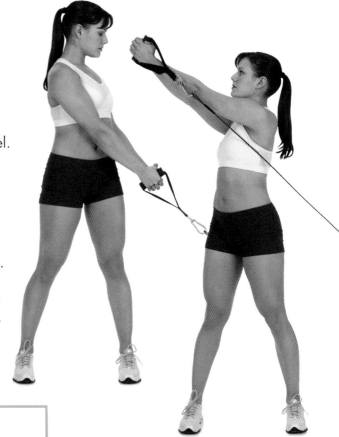

- Stand upright, twisting your torso to one side and grasping a cable handle with both hands at thigh level. Keep your arms straight.

- Pull the cable handle up across your body to your opposite shoulder. Repeat, starting on the opposite side.

- Concentrate on moving your hips and shoulders, not your arms.

HINTS

- Mimic the motion of drawing a sword by pulling the cable handle from your hip up and over one shoulder, then back down and across your body.
- Keep the motion smooth and avoid jerky movements. • Rotate through your hips and shoulders, keeping your arms straight. • Shift your feet if necessary.

STRENGTH INTENSITY	TONE INTENSITY
3 sets	3 sets
10 reps	12 reps
45 seconds rest between sets	30 seconds rest between sets

#9 BACK STRETCH 1

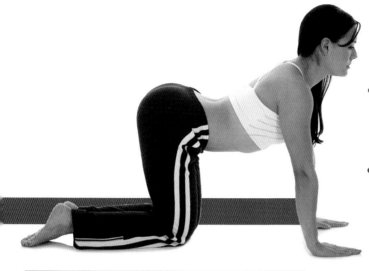

- Position yourself on all fours with your back slightly rounded.

- Round your back upward by pulling in your abdominal muscles and lifting your shoulders.

STRENGTH INTENSITY	TONE INTENSITY
Hold for 10 seconds. Repeat 3 times.	Hold for 10 seconds. Repeat 3 times.

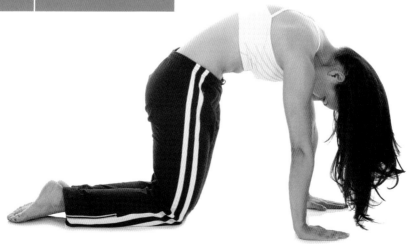

#10 HAMSTRING STRETCH 4

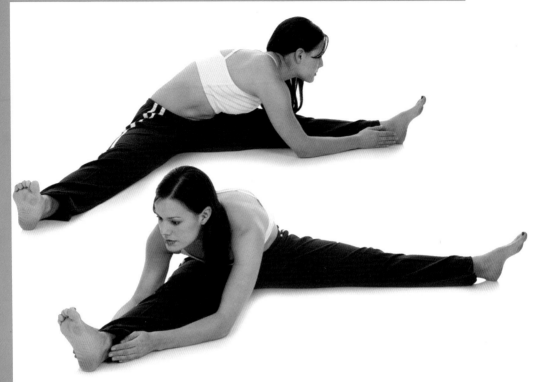

- Sit on the floor with your legs apart and straight out to the sides.

- Lean forward to one side, bringing your chest to your knee and your hands to your ankle.

- Repeat on the other side.

STRENGTH INTENSITY	TONE INTENSITY
Hold for 10 seconds. Repeat 3 times on each leg.	Hold for 10 seconds. Repeat 3 times on each leg.

#11 HIP FLEXOR STRETCH 2

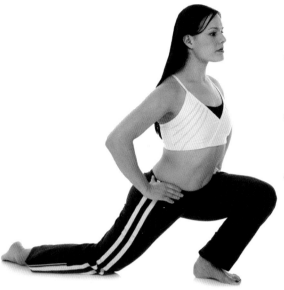

- With one knee on the floor, step slightly forward into a lunge.

- Lean into your front foot, pushing your back hip toward the floor.

- Lift your back heel to your buttocks and grasp your ankle.

STRENGTH INTENSITY	TONE INTENSITY
Hold for 10 seconds. Repeat 3 times on each leg.	Hold for 10 seconds. Repeat 3 times on each leg.

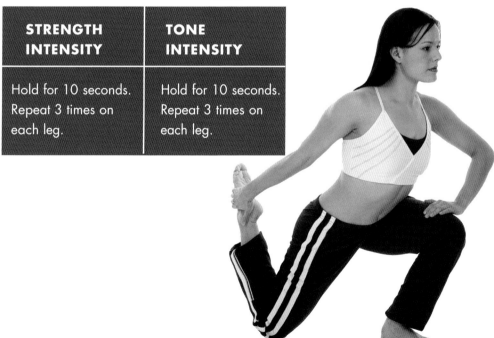

#1 DUMBBELL LUNGE

- Stand upright, holding a dumbbell in each hand by your sides, head up and looking straight forward.

- Step forward and drop your back knee toward the floor, bending both hip and knee.

- Lean slightly forward, keeping all your weight on your front foot.

- Push off the front foot to return to the starting position and repeat on the other side.

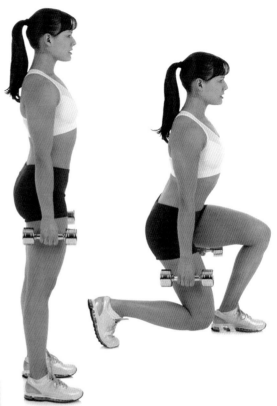

HINTS

• Keep your body weight over your front foot. • Lean forward slightly as if you were bending down to put something on the floor in front of you, being careful to maintain a flat, neutral spine. • Keep the dumbbells at the sides of your legs, not out in front.

STRENGTH INTENSITY	TONE INTENSITY
3 sets	3 sets
10 reps	12 reps
45 seconds rest between sets	30 seconds rest between sets

#2 BARBELL BENT-OVER ROW

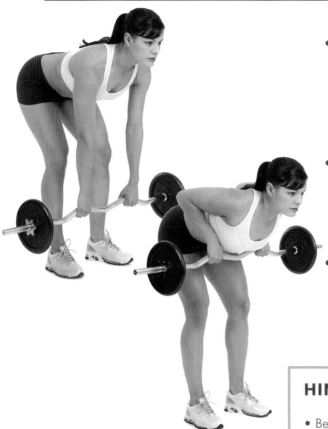

- Hold a barbell with your arms straight, as you bend forward at your waist, knees slightly bent and back flat.

- Lift the barbell up to your chest, bending your elbows and keeping them close to your sides.

- Lower the barbell to a straight-arm position, keeping your back flat.

HINTS

• Bend your knees slightly to help keep your back flat. • Don't round your back as you lower the barbell. • Pull your shoulder blades together at the top position. • Keep your head up slightly and look straight forward.

STRENGTH INTENSITY	TONE INTENSITY
3 sets	3 sets
10 reps	12 reps
45 seconds rest between sets	30 seconds rest between sets

#3 DUMBBELL DEADLIFT

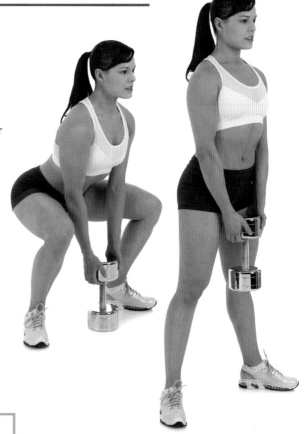

- Start in a squat position with your feet hip-width apart, your head up, and your hips low, holding a dumbbell on the floor between your feet.

- Keep your head up and look straight forward.

- Stand up, lifting the dumbbell with your arms straight and your back flat.

- Lower the dumbbell, sending your hips back and down and bending your knees.

HINTS

• Back position is very important in squatting exercises. Always maintain a neutral position. You do not want to round your lower back or over-arch it. • Keep your head up, look-ing straight forward, and keep your shoulders back. • Lower the dumbbell to the floor at the end of each rep.

STRENGTH INTENSITY	TONE INTENSITY
3 sets	3 sets
10 reps	12 reps
45 seconds rest between sets	30 seconds rest between sets

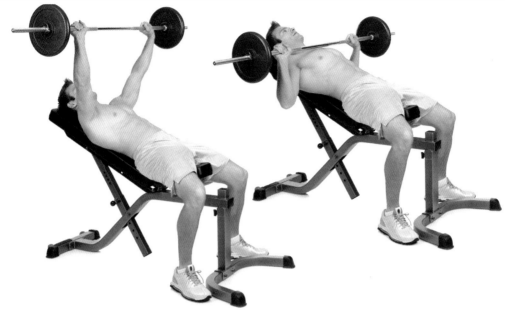

STRENGTH INTENSITY	TONE INTENSITY
3 sets	3 sets
10 reps	12 reps
45 seconds rest between sets	30 seconds rest between sets

- Lie on an incline bench holding a large barbell straight up over your chest with your arms straight and hands shoulder-width apart.

- Lower the barbell down to upper-chest level.

- Press the barbell back up to a straight-arm position.

HINTS

• Lower the barbell to your upper chest level, not your neck. • Use an even grip so your arms are centered under the barbell. • Do not bounce the barbell off your chest; instead, barely touch down before pressing back up.

#5 BARBELL PUSH PRESS

- Stand upright holding the barbell in front of you at shoulder height with your hands shoulder-width apart, elbows bent, and palms facing forward.

- Bend your hips and knees slightly and then quickly lift the barbell overhead, extending your arms and legs fully.

- Keep your back flat and stand upright throughout the exercise.

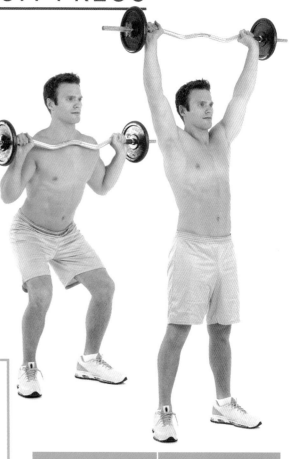

HINTS

• Keep your back flat by contracting your core muscles as you lift and push the barbell overhead. • Go through the full range of motion from shoulder level to arms fully extended overhead and back again. • As you push the barbell overhead, use your legs as much as possible, as if you were about to jump off the floor.

STRENGTH INTENSITY	TONE INTENSITY
3 sets	3 sets
10 reps	12 reps
45 seconds rest between sets	30 seconds rest between sets

#6 MEDICINE BALL TWIST

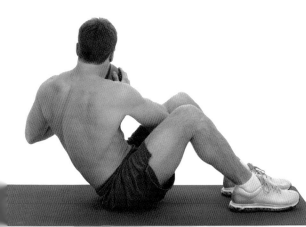

- Start in a sit-up position with your feet flat and knees bent. Hold a medicine ball at chest level.

- Twist your torso to one side, lowering the medicine ball toward the floor on that side.

- Twist your torso back to the other side.

STRENGTH INTENSITY	TONE INTENSITY
3 sets	3 sets
10 reps	12 reps
45 seconds rest between sets	30 seconds rest between sets

HINTS

• Twist through your midsection; don't just move your arms. • Turn your head and shoulders to the sides for each rep.

#7 SINGLE-LEG FRONT BRIDGE

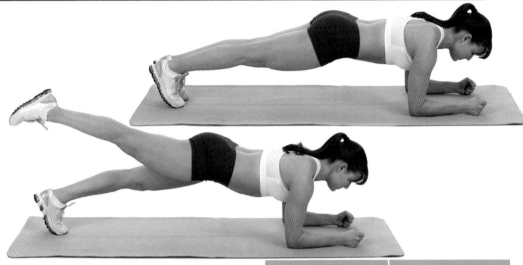

- Lie face down on a mat with your legs straight and arms tucked in by your sides.

- Lift yourself so that your weight is on your forearms and toes.

- Raise one leg off the floor, resting on one foot and your forearms.

- Try to maintain your body in a straight line, and keep your back flat.

- Hold for ten seconds, then lower yourself back to the floor.

STRENGTH INTENSITY	TONE INTENSITY
3 sets	3 sets
10 reps	12 reps
45 seconds rest between sets	30 seconds rest between sets

HINTS

• You can start in a kneeling position with your hands on the floor. • Lift your hips and hold your torso in this position throughout the exercise. • Start with your feet hip-width apart before you lift one foot off the mat. • Keep your elbows directly under your shoulders.

#8 BICYCLE CRUNCH

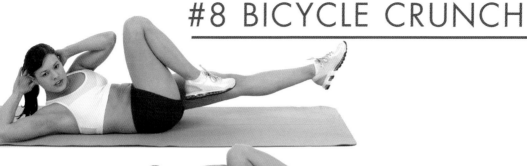

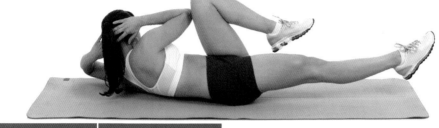

STRENGTH INTENSITY	TONE INTENSITY
3 sets	3 sets
10 reps	12 reps
45 seconds rest between sets	30 seconds rest between sets

- Lie on your back with your legs straight and your hands at the sides of your head.

- Lift your head and shoulders off the floor, bringing one knee toward your chest.

- Twist your torso, moving the opposite elbow to your knee.

- Lower your upper body and leg to the floor. Repeat, twisting to the opposite side and using your other leg.

HINTS

• Return to the down position every time before switching to the other side. • Turn your head and shoulders as you twist to each side. • Try to keep your feet off the floor throughout the exercise, but if this is too much, touch your heels to the floor.

#9 SAW TWIST

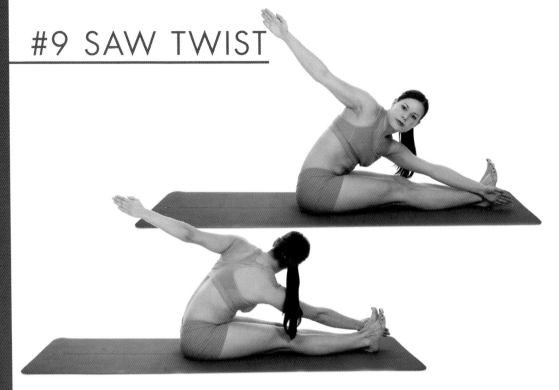

- Sit upright with your legs straight out in front, feet shoulder-width apart. Extend your arms straight out to your sides at shoulder height.

- Slowly twist your upper body to one side, stretching one hand to the opposite foot. Hold and exhale.

- Return to the upright position and twist to the opposite side.

STRENGTH INTENSITY	TONE INTENSITY
Hold for 10 seconds. Repeat 3 times on each side.	Hold for 10 seconds. Repeat 3 times on each side.

#10 BACK STRETCH 2

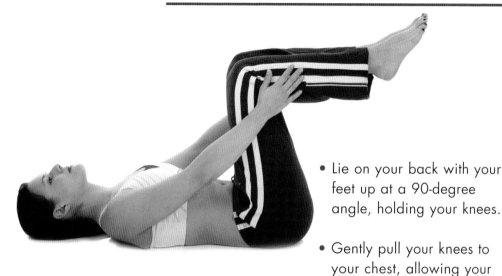

- Lie on your back with your feet up at a 90-degree angle, holding your knees.

- Gently pull your knees to your chest, allowing your lower back to round slightly.

STRENGTH INTENSITY	TONE INTENSITY
Hold for 10 seconds. Repeat 3 times.	Hold for 10 seconds. Repeat 3 times.

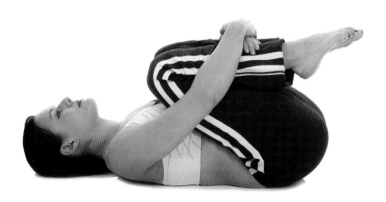

#11 QUADRICEPS STRETCH 2

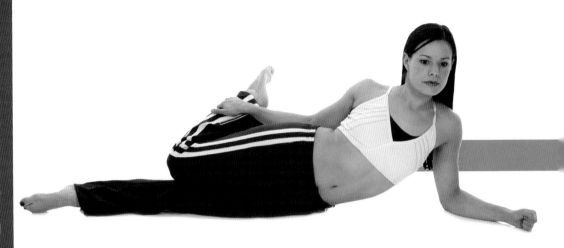

- Lie on your side with your bottom leg straight out.

- Bend your top knee, grasp your ankle, and gently pull your foot to your buttocks.

STRENGTH INTENSITY	TONE INTENSITY
Hold for 10 seconds. Repeat 3 times on each leg.	Hold for 10 seconds. Repeat 3 times on each leg.

#1 HAMSTRING STRETCH 2

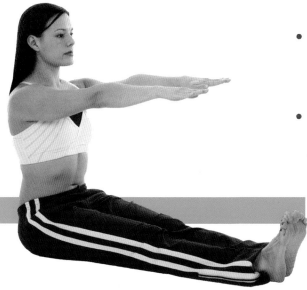

- Sit upright with both your legs and arms straight out in front of you.

- Lean forward, reaching straight arms toward your toes while keeping your legs straight.

STRENGTH INTENSITY	TONE INTENSITY
Hold for 10 seconds. Repeat 3 times.	Hold for 10 seconds. Repeat 3 times.

#2 GLUTE STRETCH 1

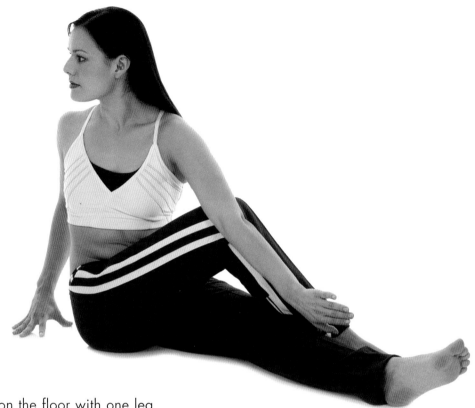

- Sit on the floor with one leg straight and the other bent and crossed to the outside of the straight leg.

- Place your opposite elbow on the outside of the bent knee.

- Gently pull your knee across your body with your elbow as you face the other side.

STRENGTH INTENSITY	TONE INTENSITY
Hold for 10 seconds. Repeat 3 times on each leg.	Hold for 10 seconds. Repeat 3 times on each leg.

#3 HIP FLEXOR STRETCH 1

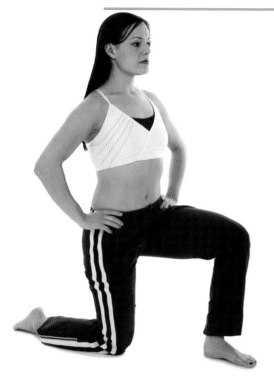

- With one knee on the floor, position the other slightly forward with your knee bent.

- Shift your weight onto your front foot, pushing your back hip toward the floor.

STRENGTH INTENSITY	TONE INTENSITY
Hold for 10 seconds. Repeat 3 times on each leg.	Hold for 10 seconds. Repeat 3 times on each leg.

#4 BACK STRETCH 1

- Position yourself on all fours with your back slightly rounded into a dip.

- Lift and round your back by pulling in your abdominal muscles and lifting your shoulders.

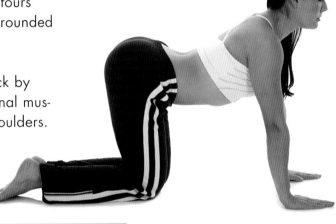

STRENGTH INTENSITY	TONE INTENSITY
Hold for 10 seconds. Repeat 3 times.	Hold for 10 seconds. Repeat 3 times.

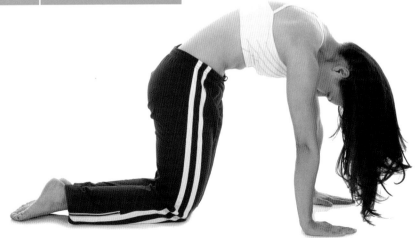

#5 UPWARD DOG

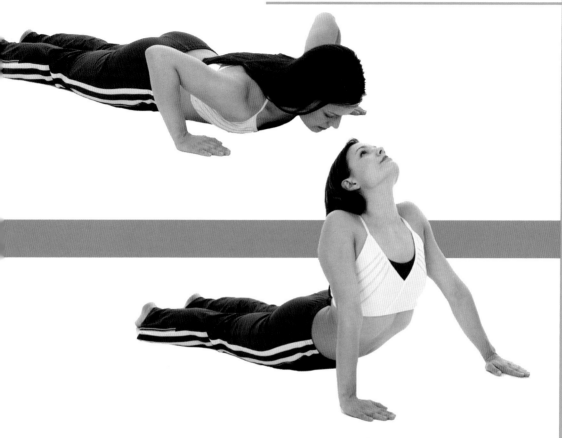

STRENGTH INTENSITY	TONE INTENSITY
Hold for 10 seconds. Repeat 3 times.	Hold for 10 seconds. Repeat 3 times.

- Lie face down with your hands by your shoulders and your elbows bent.

- Push up your upper body, arching your back and keeping your hips and legs on the floor.

#6 QUADRICEPS STRETCH 1

- Stand upright on one leg, bending the other leg at the knee and lifting your heel to your buttocks.

- Grasp your ankle with one hand and gently pull your foot farther for a deeper stretch.

#7 CALF STRETCH 1

- Stand upright, bracing yourself against a wall with your back leg straight out behind and your front leg slightly bent.

- Keeping your back foot flat on the floor, shift your body weight forward onto your front leg.

STRENGTH INTENSITY	TONE INTENSITY
Hold for 10 seconds. Repeat 3 times on each leg.	Hold for 10 seconds. Repeat 3 times on each leg.

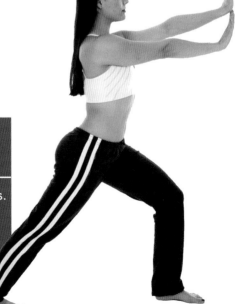

#8 LATERAL STRETCH

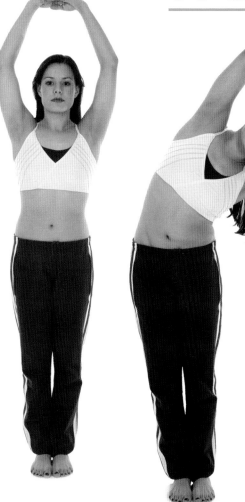

- Stand upright with your feet together and your arms straight overhead, hands clasped.

- Lean to one side, moving your arms laterally.

- Move back to the upright position, then switch sides.

STRENGTH INTENSITY	TONE INTENSITY
Hold for 10 seconds. Repeat 3 times on each side.	Hold for 10 seconds. Repeat 3 times on each side.

#1 HAMSTRING STRETCH 1

- Lie on your back with your arms at your sides. Lift one leg.

- Grasp your extended ankle or calf with one hand and gently pull your foot closer for a deeper stretch.

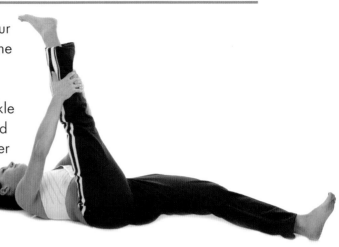

#2 GLUTE STRETCH 2

- Lie on your back with your legs straight.

- Bend one knee and grasp it with the opposite hand.

- Use the hand on your knee to pull it across your body and down toward the floor.

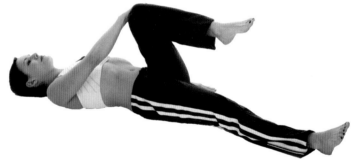

STRENGTH INTENSITY	TONE INTENSITY
Hold for 10 seconds. Repeat 3 times on each leg.	Hold for 10 seconds. Repeat 3 times on each leg.

#3 HIP FLEXOR STRETCH 2

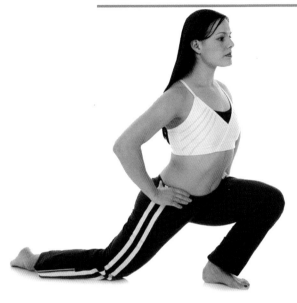

- With one knee on the floor, position the other slightly forward with your knee bent.

- Shift your weight onto your front foot, pushing your back hip toward the floor.

- Raise your back heel to your buttocks, grasping at the ankle.

STRENGTH INTENSITY	TONE INTENSITY
Hold for 10 seconds. Repeat 3 times on each leg.	Hold for 10 seconds. Repeat 3 times on each leg.

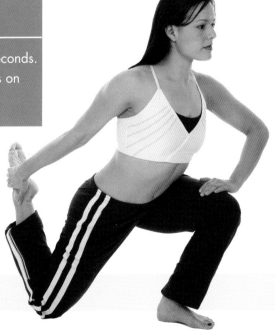

STRETCH SEQUENCE 2

#4 BACK STRETCH 2

- Lie on your back with your feet up at a 90-degree angle, holding your knees.

- Gently pull your knees to your chest, allowing your lower back to round slightly.

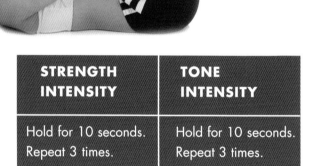

STRENGTH INTENSITY	TONE INTENSITY
Hold for 10 seconds. Repeat 3 times.	Hold for 10 seconds. Repeat 3 times.

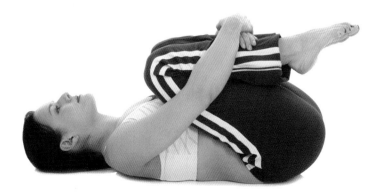

#5 BACK STRETCH 3

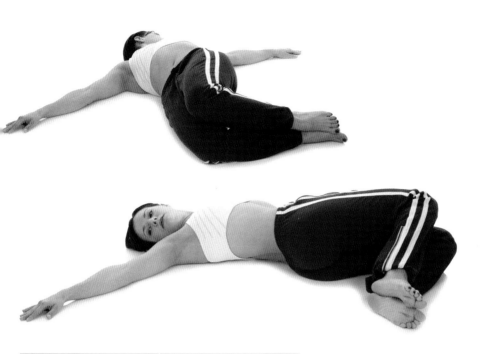

STRENGTH INTENSITY	TONE INTENSITY
Hold for 10 seconds. Repeat 3 times on each side.	Hold for 10 seconds. Repeat 3 times on each side.

- Lie flat on your back with your knees bent and feet together and your arms straight out to the sides at shoulder height.

- Lower your knees to touch the floor on one side as you turn your head to the other side.

- Repeat on the opposite side, switching both your legs and head position.

#6 QUADRICEPS STRETCH 2

- Lie on your side with your bottom leg straight out.

- Bend your top knee, grasp your ankle, and gently pull your foot to your buttocks.

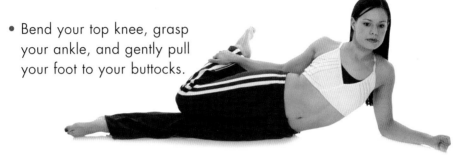

#7 CALF STRETCH 2

- Stand upright, bracing yourself against a wall with your front foot on a dumbbell or an incline block and your leg straight.

- Shift your body weight forward into your front leg.

- Be sure to keep your foot at an incline.

STRENGTH INTENSITY	TONE INTENSITY
Hold for 10 seconds. Repeat 3 times on each leg.	Hold for 10 seconds. Repeat 3 times on each leg.

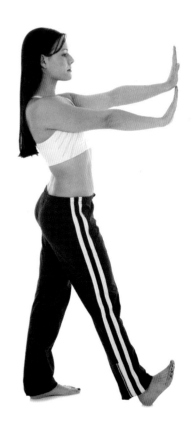

#8 PECTORAL STRETCH WITH SWISS BALL

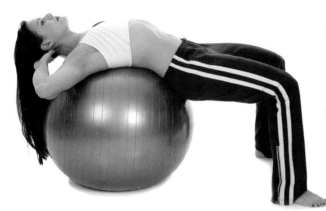

- Lie with your mid-back on a Swiss ball and your hands at the sides of your head.

- Roll back slightly on the ball and extend your arms overhead.

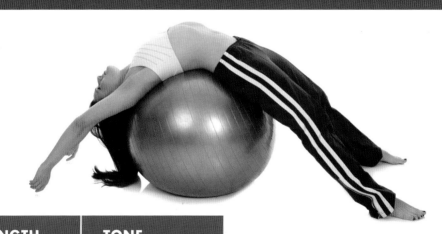

STRENGTH INTENSITY	TONE INTENSITY
Hold for 10 seconds. Repeat 3 times.	Hold for 10 seconds. Repeat 3 times.

INDEX

Back pain
  exercise helping, 4, 5
  preventing, 5
  spinal anatomy/function and, 6
  symptoms and causes, 4
Bar
  Hip Abduction with Bar, 72
  Modified Self-Row, 82
  Self Row with Bar, 115
  Straight Bar Hip Adduction, 94
Barbells
  Back Squat, 114
  Bench Press, 84, 117
  Bent-Over Row, 137
  Deadlift, 125
  Incline Bench Press, 139
  Overhead Press, 107
  Pullover, 128
  Push Press, 140
  Upright Row, 129
Bench work. See also Barbells;
  Dumbbells
  Bench Dip, 42
  Bench Toe Taps, 17
  Raised-Feet Bench Dip, 106
  Reverse Hyperextension, 131
Bodyweight and body-only exercises.
  See also Stretching
  Alternating Bridge, 109
  Alternating Flyer, 44
  Bicycle Crunch, 35, 143
  Crunch, 43, 64
  Deadbug, 23
  Feet-Up Crunch, 53
  Flutter Kicks, 88
  Flyer, 24, 130
  Front Bridge, 34, 76
  Glute Bridge, 41
  Glute Bridge March, 61
  Glute Kickback, 83
  Jackknife, 77
  Kneeling Push-Up, 22
  Lower Body Twist, 25
  Lunge, 59
  Oblique Bridge, 55, 99
  Oblique Crunch, 75
  Pelvic Lift, 21
  Pelvic Tilt, 33
  Push-Up, 62
  Quad Flyer, 54, 87
  Reverse Crunch, 86
  Reverse Lunge, 29

Side Bridge with Abduction, 121
Side Lunge, 49
Single-Leg Front Bridge, 142
Squat, 19
Twisting Crunch, 97
Book, how it works, 8
Cable systems
  about: substitute for, 11
  Cable Twist, 45
  Close-Grip Pulldown, 20, 71
  High-Low Chop, 110
  Hip Abduction, 51
  Hip Extension, 31
  Low-High Chop, 132
  Seated Row, 40, 93
  Standing Row, 104
  Wide Grip Pulldown, 50
Dumbbells
  Bench Press, 32
  Bilateral Bent-Over Row, 126
  Deadlift, 39, 138
  Fly, 73
  Front Raise, 118
  Incline Bench Press, 52
  Lateral Raise, 85
  Lunge, 136
  Overhead Press, 63
  Prone Bench Row, 30
  Prone Dumbbell Back Delt Row, 96
  Pullover, 95
  Reverse Lunge, 92
  Row Over Bench, 60
  Side Bend, 66
  Side Lunge, 116
  Split Squat, 70
  Squat, 103
  Step-Up, 81, 127
  Stiff-Leg Deadlift, 105
  Upright Row, 74
Equipment, 11. See also specific equip-
  ment
Exercise, benefits of, 4, 5, 7
Level 1, Workout 1, 19–28
Level 1, Workout 2, 29–38
Level 1, Workout 3, 39–48
Level 1, Workout 4, 49–58
Level 2, Workout 1, 59–69
Level 2, Workout 2, 70–80
Level 2, Workout 3, 81–91
Level 2, Workout 4, 92–102
Level 3, Workout 1, 103–113
Level 3, Workout 2, 114–124

Level 3, Workout 3, 125–135
Level 3, Workout 4, 136–146
Medicine Ball Twist, 119, 141
Safety precautions, 9–10
Spinal anatomy/function, 6
Starting out, 11
Stretching. See also Swiss ball
  Back Stretch 1, 27, 79, 133, 150
  Back Stretch 2, 47, 101, 145, 156
  Back Stretch 3, 122, 157
  Calf Stretch 1, 152
  Calf Stretch 2, 158
  Glute Stretch 1, 26, 80, 148
  Glute Stretch 2, 36, 102, 154
  Glute Stretch 3, 46
  Hamstring Stretch 1, 38, 100, 123,
    154
  Hamstring Stretch 2, 56, 91, 112,
    147
  Hamstring Stretch 3, 67
  Hamstring Stretch 4, 78, 134
  Hip Flexor Stretch 1, 48, 69, 113,
    149
  Hip Flexor Stretch 2, 58, 89, 135,
    155
  Lateral Stretch, 68, 153
  Pectoral Stretch, 90, 159
  Quadriceps Stretch 1, 124, 152
  Quadriceps Stretch 2, 146, 158
  Saw Twist, 144
  Single Leg Stretch, 28, 57
  Upward Dog, 37, 111, 151
Stretching Sequence 1, 147–153
Stretching Sequence 2, 154–159
Swiss ball
  Elbow Bridge, 120
  Pectoral Stretch, 90, 159
  Reverse Extension, 108
  T, 98
  Y, 65
Warming up and cooling down, 10,
  12. See also Stretching references
Warm-ups
  Bench Toe Taps, 17
  Bodyweight Squats, 16
  Elliptical Machine (or Crosstrainer),
    13
  Jog in Place, 15
  Jumping Jacks, 18
  Twisting Punch, 14
Workouts. See Level references